By being a vegan for the past six years, the writer wanted to make the idea of veganism attainable. Noting the same thought trails the writer experienced when first starting the diet, the reader will feel more comfortable in trying the diet. And also let out some chuckles.

Victoria Levitt

SHIRLEY TRIES A NEW DIET

AUSTIN MACAULEY PUBLISHERS™

LONDON • CAMBRIDGE • NEW YORK • SHARJAH

A CIP catalogue record for this title is available from the British Library.

ISBN 9781528990608 (Paperback)
ISBN 9781528990615 (ePub e-book)

www.austinmacauley.com

First Published (2020)
Austin Macauley Publishers Ltd
25 Canada Square
Canary Wharf
London
E14 5LQ

To my mum, dad and auntie Jill

Chapter 1

I've counted seven months and fourteen days since I've finished being with Claude as I thought it would be for the best life in some way. I endured all the stereotypical things to do, like eat tubs of ice cream and crying myself to sleep but I got bored of it, so now need something else that I can have and get into. First thoughts sounded easy, but I just sat looking how other people walked hand in hand down the street. This period only lasted a couple of months, but the large advertisement placed on the nearby billboard caught my attention. It mentioned 'Online Dating'. This could be my fairy-tale moment. I will forget about my ex-boyfriend and find another love. My online being implored me to be creative and very relatable as well as being very single. Completing this task meant I could go up the romantic ladder to reach perfect love happiness. When creating a profile name, I thought it best to use the name of my dearly loved toy sheep who I've had for many years. She cuddled me through the sleepless nights after becoming single, so I hoped Shirley Sheep could serve as my online dating profile name.

Deciding this online mask, I began my whirlwind of the dating world. I stumbled into a new beau when I thought it would have been happily ever after. Unfortunately, he turned out to be a fraud and I ended up being just myself. Especially when Claude, my devilishly handsome new boyfriend, ended up by telling me excuses like how he was doing 'extra time at work'. When the number of him being away from home reached six nights, I thought it was best to be doubtful even though I never heard any gossip recounting his 24 hours away from home. I was aware some couples on farms had split because of courting other ovine, but I really didn't feel that would happen between me and Claude. I chose Claude because of him ranking highly on my relationship quota list and finding any likeminded someone who showed no sign of playing away. He didn't even notice another female on our dates. I don't think.

I thought that my avatar of Shirley could continue for longer, especially as I was a singleton, something I didn't realise, lasted too long. The local farmers had given me a role at a nearby farm and judging from my past work experience, the new position could be taken up whenever I liked.

Sure, there was an influx of new ovine turning over each month. Becoming friends with any of them in the flock was never a strong point of my character. I was after all, in the mindset of being in a relationship. Thanks to the worthless ram, Claude, I didn't bother with any of the good-looking males. My best friend, Charlene, thought it could be helped if I joined a club of some sort. I tutted at her, but nothing has been produced for me to choose from. I love Charlene to bits but was immensely jealous of her happy attitude to life. She has helped me when selecting the best dating site. So surely, she can help me post the whole dating malarkey around this farm.

Charlene looked scared when I trotted over to her. I tried my best not to have a smug knowing look, but this was difficult, and I blurted out the words, "I've done what you told me to do, but he really wasn't interested!" The words were difficult to say but I did feel rejoiced I'd said them. Charlene was a scared sheep and I had made it an internal rule to not shout at her.

I didn't mean to create moods of pressure, but I did add looks of need with my head bent at an angle, Charlene looked at me and she did same thing I have given her multiple times: a big eye roll. I loudly grumbled to make her aware of my feelings about her doing that. I thought it best to say something to really get to a point but settled on, "Have you got any other ideas for me to do?"

Events in my life were to stand in a field and not do anything at all. Was Claude really the best of my love interests? I stood wistfully, looking at the herd in my field, this way I looked intelligent. Thankfully, Charlene bounded over and broke my thinking moments. Something a quizzical look would gain an answer. To keep her keen to speak, I raised my eyebrows and widened my eyes. These motions have previously worked on getting the latest farmyard gossip. Charlene was never a fast answering sheep, this was something I got used to after three years of sharing a field with her, so I learnt the best methods of coaxing an answer. My best choice was to pre-empt an answer but get it so badly wrong that she would jump in to correct me.

"What are you thinking about? Your eyes are moving around quickly without focussing on anything. You've told me in the past that happens when you're thinking, so as you haven't said anything for the past minute, I thought I would ask you. If it is a personal matter, you know I would keep quiet."

I didn't make a sound to answer her question, in fact in the past, I have left Charlene answerless, but for today I could see an answer quite useful. I do want to meet this sporty ram and Charlene would probably know his exact location.

"Well, Charlene, I've been thinking about the words you told me earlier and about meeting sporty sheep again and what we could do."

Charlene's face instantly beamed with a smile and even accentuated her happy mood by clapping her hooves. These were actions I never enjoyed; in fact I would label it as selfish because I wasn't sharing her mood. I let out a small laugh to let her know I too, was happy, not as happy as she was, judging by the over the top show she performed. I thought it best to offer her a question, one where she could show off her knowledge of ovine locations. In the past, Charlene had offered me the lists of the new flocks and their locations, she wouldn't be offended if I pried her knowledge once again.

"Where do you think sporty sheep actually are? What farm exactly and whereabouts do they graze?"

My question was completely answerable for her and I didn't fear remaining answerless.

"Well, Shirley, one of the sporty lot is a sheep called William and he's a Border Leicester stock. They're quite agile so no wonder you call him sporty! I'm not sure where his boyfriend is but can give you information soon. Next week? I can give you more information, especially regarding your first conversation with him."

Charlene finished her sentence with a cheeky wink. I made my objection of her wink and told her to go off to her contacts to find more information.

I followed Charlene's instructions to track down this 'William' and started by entering the nearby farm. There was not a wish of mine that wanted to set her off being exceptionally happy because of how she behaved last night. With all her hoof clapping and loud screaming. I thought it best to catch her eye and smile. That plan was to be held in utmost silence, something I hoped Charlene would equal and lessen her tone. We were after all in a different farm so should respect all the other guys grazing. I mean, they were working after all.

It didn't take long for the presumed shrieking and shouting to occur as Charlene neared.

"SHIRLEY!"

I became instantly interested in what she had to say as I was due to pass her, being on my route back to my farm's original location. Probably in thirty seconds but I didn't want to rush my lunch break so lessoned my pace and just hoped I wasn't met with an excited ewe squally, uselessly for no point. I came across exactly that.

"Hey there, Shirley! How are you! Why are you here? Did you get lost?"

I gave her about ten seconds to calm down from her initial excitement. If she was going to deliver me anymore words, I wanted her to deliver it succinctly and timely. I thought it best to speak in a calm manner, so I straightened my wool around my head and took a deep breath.

"So, you know how much I love drama in these fields, right?"

I couldn't argue against that so just gave a gentle nod. I was still awaiting what she's done to cause her embarrassment and rosy hue. I thought it best to ask a straightforward question.

"What have you been doing today? Have you been doing any exercise because your cheeks are a bit red?"

There, I said it, so Charlene needs to answer. I have been called rude for speaking my mind but for this case it's justified.

"No, Shirley! I haven't been doing any exercise, I just wandered across the fields to meet a ram who you might be interested in. We've been told off for taking too long for lunches, so I skipped down the pathways to come back. I know I need to work on my fitness, but I can understand why my cheeks are glowing!"

This still didn't answer much of my initial question, so I thought it best to repeat it.

"Who did you 'wander' into?"

I thought it best to be specific, after all she ploughs me for information daily about lots of frivolous stuff. My favourite choice of questions were about the fashion and which celebrity wore the best tops. Charlene once took me shopping and acknowledged the season's fashion in every store that we passed. I didn't hold any worry about any question I've asked. I do have a worry about how long she takes to answer a simple question.

"Well, I visited Fawcett fields to see if there was anyone worth knowing."

And I had to endure another uninteresting bout of silence, so I decided to quicken things up,

"Who did you meet?"

The same question but asked in a different way. She must have understood what I was saying. I couldn't ask her another time because she would think of me being rude. Which is, of course, what I had no worry about doing.

"I met Steve. He looked very healthy and good looking and is going out with your guy, William."

I didn't want to waste time pointing out the 'your guy' comment because I knew exactly who she meant. It was Mr Sporty.

The possibilities were exciting to me, I could make two new friends if I played my cards right. I could woo William with my good personality and then get introduced to his boy-friend with glorious acclaim. Making friends would be easy.

"Thank you for your answer. I'm looking forward to ac-tually meeting Mr Sporty one day soon."

I threw in a tasteless wink to make her happy, I was pre-dicting a snarl of laughter to occur after that.

"Oh gosh! Yes, Shirley! We must meet Sporty and then make him introduce us to Steve! Apparently, they're a good couple and always up for a drink. Something you're good at."

And then it was my chance to blush. Charlene hasn't been on this farm for too long, well, under three years so she's rel-atively a newbie. Not long enough for her to make a sweeping statement about my alcohol consumption. I didn't cause any-thing truly negative to happen because of my over drinking, but yes, I have fallen over several times when Mr Grigio got scary but nothing to write home about. Did she really think it was something I was good at? As if I could have easily whipped back at her by saying she was really good at breath-ing. I didn't want to get in to the severity of verbs, so I changed the subject.

"What are you up to tomorrow, Charlene? Fancy a Wil-liam hunt?"

That was one question I didn't have to wait long for an answer as I was met with a host of squeals and shouts of YES!

So, we planned to make our way over to the bottom of our field at lunchtime to see if William was about. We planned to stay there for fifteen minutes before leaving for the next field.

"My sources have told me that William has moved to a new grazing location. It is in Fawcett fields but now closer to the main gate. This is something we must be aware of; do you copy that, Shirley?"

I hated when others used army type talk to converse with me. It's as though they want to belittle me. I recognise I'm a strong character and frequently use it on others, so for now I let it slide and mumbled,

"Copied."

No salute was added after saying that, but I felt a dose of poetic license was granted to me. Charlene enjoyed that and returned the salute action. My feelings of excitement began to grow from that moment. We could have a fun time tomorrow and meeting Mr Sporty/William could actually be a fun experience.

"What are you planning on saying to William when you meet him?"

That was quite a question from Charlene, one that I realised needed more preparation for. If I came face-to-face with him, I needed to run through a set of questions to ask. I thought it best to use the questioner as a source of ideas. The best way of getting these ideas was to directly ask her and appear worrisome with creased forehead lines.

"What do you think I should say?"

I praised myself on my delivery of the question, it oozed a sense of utter neediness.

"Well, I suppose you need to chat about something you're quite familiar with. Maybe a film you've recently seen? You could chat about the main character? Or you could chat about TV? At the end of the day you could always rely upon the weather because everybody does that."

Drilling into Charlene's idea bank proved useful and I had enough material to train myself to work with. The plan needed to have some sort of ending, how long should I be chatting to William for? I think a question to Charlene was needed.

"So, if I chat with William, how long should I chat to him for? Are we going out for a drink after?"

Charlene sighed and tilted her head, I think she was performing a thinking pose. I hoped.

"Of course, we should go for a drink! I'm not sure where though. After finding out if he's available to do something later, you could ask him, where's the best place to drink?"

Of course, that's the perfect line to say to him, I was annoyed I hadn't thought of it immediately.

"I'm going to head off for the day, Shirley, see you tomorrow and make sure you smell nice for tomorrow's meet!"

The shelf that holds multiple perfumes to select my odour for the day proved useful as I opted for 'White Linen' to really give myself an aura of friendliness. Something that I thought William would appreciate as he looked really smart when I briefly saw him. He probably smelled good, but I was too far away to really get a sniff. From the initial 'hi' with him I gained the opinion that he was a sheep who was easily ticking off the things you say in the CV like presentable, time conscious and self-aware.

Charlene was late coming in to work, but I kept my annoyance down as I didn't want anything that could intervene with my new odour, having a rush of sweat around my body could damage the newly spritzed on smell. I had to recollect what the plan was as I became ever more dubious with each minute of waiting. As soon as I started thinking about a plan, breaking off from the created plan and trotting off down the road to Fawcett fields farm, Charlene emerged daintily skipping up the hill to our usual grazing spot. It didn't take long to notice the amount of effort she had spent on her face with it having heavy eye powder and strong cheek blusher.

Charlene only told me to put an odour on which I duly followed. I honestly haven't a clue as to why she is so dolled up, normally we let each other know exactly how we are preparing ourselves for a night out. This needs to be discussed when she is near me.

"Hey, Shirley! As there's a possibility of us going out to the pub if William wants to go, I thought it best to spruce myself up beforehand."

So that was quite an answer to my thinking about her looking so glamorous. I felt annoyed at myself for not putting any makeup on, in fact reasonably naked. One thing was sure; I did smell nice.

"Is it all right if you could help me put on make-up at lunch before we cross over to Fawcett farm? I want to look as good as you."

I gave a smiling face and brought my hoofs together in the action of symbolising a prayer. I thought this action was best as I became worried Charlene would forget our plan created yesterday. She had gone off-piste with her make-up appearance so she could go off-piste again, so I needed to make her aware of the lines.

"Yeah sure, darling! Have you got mascara? I think a heavy coating could go a long way, so I'd be happy to do that to you at lunch. You won't forget to ask William if it's all right to go with him."

This was a stupid thing to say. I had spent the night running over the topics I should start with; films, TV and songs. If I got desperate, I would rely upon the weather. After hearing my lunch time plans confirmed, I felt at ease. Hopefully, William will be available to come for a drink tonight with us, if he's not, then I will ask Charlene to come to the pub with me. This is something we've done many times and perhaps led to her thinking I 'liked to drink'. I'll ask Charlene to give me the most accurate estimate of Mr Sporty's location when she was next free to talk. After she had helped with my make-up.

Both I and Charlene went to the closest barn and she mimicked being an A-list make-up artist and told me where to look. I abided by these instructions and held a genuine hope I will finish the session looking like a model.

The chat was friendly and helped with the planning of where I should go next to meet this William again. We were both certain that he would be down the field by the sheds as that was where I saw him first, if not, I was to go to the next adjacent farm where he probably will be because his boyfriend was somewhere around there. When everything was achieved, we looked at each other and nodded which was followed by a grin. Charlene did a superb job on my makeup, so much that I whole heartedly congratulated her. This was a rare action from me. The last time I did such a thing was to say something to a marathon runner last year because everyone else said something congratulatory, so I joined in. Peer pressure is not something I want to do, but I'm aware it can aid social interactions sometimes.

Off I trotted out of the barn then, beckoned Charlene to join me, to which she did. I felt better when she was by my side, meeting William was a big task for me. Not in a romantic way, but I really wanted for him to be my friend, all of the herd knows of him and holds him in high standards. As I've said, I never bow to peer pressure but for this one time, I will. I should practise my introductory lines again.

"There he is, Shirl!" exclaimed Charlene.

I thought her shouting was a bit over the top as he stood only nine metres away.

"Yes, thank you, Charlene, let's trot over together?"

When we stood face to face with him, he unleashed another of his gleaming white toothed smiles, just like he did to me. No wonder, I thought he went off to a model photoshoot, his grin was impressive, coupled with his bright-blue eyes; he could only be a part-time model. I took a moment to fully appreciate his stature, but Charlene interrupted my silent moment.

"Hi there, are you called William?"

I really hoped he was or else Charlene's knowledge of who's who on the farm was false. Thankfully, he was as he immediately looked up into Charlene's eyes and smiled to say, "That's right! I'm William! And you are?"

I'll be amazed if he could recognise me, but I'll step away from the introductions.

"My name is Charlene and I'm here with my friend, Shirley, who you might recognise."

She didn't need to use her hands and display me like an auction piece whilst saying that.

William nodded and pointed at me before saying,

"YES! I saw you briefly the other day! I just assumed you were a scout!"

This was my chance to take the overly cheerful reins from Charlene,

"I told you he was a model didn't I, Charlene? I thought you didn't believe me. Models probably have lots of scouts working with them. Is that right, William?"

I broke my silence to enjoy a 'I told you so' moment, something I enjoy doing.

William looked up to me and nodded with a grin.

"Yeah, I quite often get different sheep coming to look at me, usually they give me a contact card, but you didn't, Shirley. That's all right, what are you two ewes doing tonight?"

He stole one of the lines I was going to use on him, but I won't be offended because Charlene was eager to bleat.

"We are both free tonight and wondered if you wanted to do something with us? I'm sure the Red Lion down the road will have enough space for us if you fancy going?"

From the end of her sentence, William let off a happy affirmative sound and quickly said, "Yeah! Let's do that. Is it all right if my boyfriend joins us? He's quite quiet and won't be annoying or anything, it's just that I told him I was free tonight and he suggested going to the pub."

I and Charlene looked at each other with faces full of giddy happiness and in almost unison we shouted, "Yes, of course, he can come!"

Charlene broke off to show off her farm contacts list.

"Is Steve his name? I think it is, but I just wanted to be sure."

William gave a coy look and smiled followed by lots of nodding. I guessed he was excited, so I wanted to continue his happy energy by asking, "So how long have you two been going out? A long time? Or is a recent thing?"

I have a habit of answering questions I have posed so it will be interesting to hear his reaction. Although my team couldn't help herself but speak, so I needed to listen to Charlene's input before I heard William's answer.

"So, William has been going out with Steve for about a year and a half? They met at a farm near Southampton I think."

As she spoke, I watched William's reactions and nodding. Charlene was an excellent researcher; something she is well aware of. I smiled at her as if to emit feelings of pride. It took vast amounts to deliver her findings like that. Professional make up didn't have to be her only other option for work, professional research jobs could bring in money if she needed it. I thought it best to speed up our entrance to the pub.

"So guys, when are we going? Let's get the best four-seater table, I think it gets busy on a Friday!"

Simultaneously, the pair who I was speaking with, stood up and grabbed their coat and bags to walk out to the exit. It was quite a challenge to match their location from my resting position. Thankfully, I reached them before the doors of the pub opened. William smiled at us both then asked,

"What are you wanting to drink?"

We were both astounded by this and squealed our orders. I thought it was appropriate to find the best seating for us all, I did think about where Steve would want us to sit, but I just settled on one table in the middle of the room. I could really imagine us all sitting here.

Chapter 2

Both me and Charlene placed ourselves on the four-seater table and made ourselves known of our location to William who was busy with our drink order. This gave us good time to inspect the pub's interior and where we thought the herd will be seated. The arch ceiling covering would probably attract the males, those who thought they were cool, as well as the coolest ewes but we recognised we weren't cool enough so will probably stick here on this table. After the landscape deduction, William came, bearing drinks.

After sitting down and cheers were toasted, William looked as if he was desperately searching out of the large window by the door and searched for his phone in his bag. After a moment, he sighed and toasted us again. I allowed him an eye roll as I would do the same if my boyfriend hadn't have turned up by this time. As Charlene and William were busy chatting, I took a glance to look over at the bar's new customer arrival who had beckoned the member of staff and was pointing at different items on the plastic menu. The bar newbie nodded a lot, then grabbed his wallet to pay for something. As he spun around, I noticed he was a very good-looking ram, someone who I hoped to talk with and get to know. By almighty luck, this gentle ram trotted up to our table and punched William jokingly before crouching down to whisper something in his ear. I thought he must have been Steve, but he went to sit down at the end of the table. Something, I thought, was odd for a couple to do such a thing. Whether I was holding an extreme facial expression or not, William loudly shouted, "He's not my boyfriend guys, just a friend who I get along with, I'm not sure where Steve is."

I really felt for him as we had been sitting for over thirty minutes, waiting for Steve to join us. It made me wonder if Steve was keen on his boyfriend, to be honest. I tutted at myself for holding such an opinion. It didn't take much longer before Steve arrived and gave William a quick smooch, something I was deeply jealous of. I decided to cast a view down the table to the new arrival who was announced as William's friend. He was still remarkably good looking, so I was happy to just sit and appreciate the exquisite facial structure of him.

Steve after his embrace enquired to the table if anyone wanted a drink. I looked at Charlene and we both nodded. Charlene knew what she had to do and ordered our drinks, a cheeky wink that I offered was more than enough to say thank you.

When my wine arrived, I just checked whether William's friend was still there. I was very glad I did, as he looked up and we made eye contact. Wow, to get an all symmetrical view of his face was far superior to my earlier sitting position. I need to chat with William about him, he could be gay and completely off my radar. Or even worse, married.

The night trundled on and rounds of drinks were had. The conversation topics were varied but mostly focussed on what areas I had trained myself to remember to speak to William, or Mr Sporty, as I remembered him. It seemed like a pointless act as we quite happily sat here doing the aim, we most wanted. Hopefully, I didn't use up much brain juice in doing so. When I'd finished looking at Steve and wanted to join the table's conversation, I was thrilled to hear they had moved on to the topic of television.

"Did anyone watch TV last night? It was apparently in the papers today that Ofcom rules were broken. Yeh the two main characters on that romantic show said things to each other that were illegal."

There, I said something abiding by my self-imposed conversational topics. I was awaiting this line to deliver. It was gratefully received as the table was ablaze with lines of "I can't believe he said that!" "Why did them both do that?" as well as "no wonder the programme got in trouble!"

It wouldn't surprise me if another group carried on with this topic due to its volume. I felt smug regarding my initial start of this conversation. What's the other topic I wanted to chat to William about? To lure him to going to the pub with me and Charlene, It seemed a pointless thing to do as he was just down the table. I won't mention films even though I'd undoubtedly be smug. Regardless of what I say, probably best if I ask about his mate sitting down the table who I've been gazing at since talking. When I prepared myself to speak to William about films, there was a sudden shout of, "Have you seen the last film with Cameron Diaz?"

Thanks Charlene, I'm very appreciative of your conversational input but I really want to discuss William's friend who's sitting there. He looks gorgeous by the way if you haven't seen him.

"William! Who's the guy who's sitting there?"

William looked up at his mate and raised his eyebrows and smiled.

I smiled and looked at his mate, a frequent stance I've had for most of this evening.

I looked at William and gave an encouraging smile. I checked if Charlene was aware of me talking to William about this, of course she was, and I gave her a smile.

"Oh! That's Richard, he's great. Do you like him, eh?"

Charlene looked like she was going to say something, but I was dubious if she would say anything that could delay me talking with Richard.

She raised her head. "Oh, Richard. Is he the guy that's been with an ewe for like a couple of years?"

I looked intently at William's mouth hoping that it wasn't true.

"Oh yes, Richard has been going out with his girlfriend for ages but I'm not sure if they are still together."

That pricked my ears up, that's the biggest batch of hope I've had for a long time. I think I will speak again now, "So when can I meet this Richard?"

The wait for an answer could only have been a matter of seconds but I was joyful when William gave me a positive response.

"Well, I'm not sure if he's single yet, Shirley."

Charlene jumped in to enquire about their relationship status by saying, "From what I've heard, his girlfriend was going to go off with someone else, sorry, Shirley, I didn't realise you liked him so much."

I needed to give a stern reply to counteract Charlene's happiness.

"Well, I didn't know I liked him until he joined us on our table. If he was around, I definitely would have positioned my grazing position better to start a conversation with him." I gave a small tut to Charlene to myself. I thought it best to re-join my gazing some more.

"If you really want, I can say something to Richard but I'm not sure if this would be best as he might instantly dismiss you without giving you a fair break."

Well, I can deal with this and work with Charlene as to where and what I should do going forward. Charlene was smiling to herself where she leaped up after coming across an idea, something that I am very aware of after all these years.

"Oh! Wasn't he going to change his diet or something?" She looked across at William for an answer. William smiled at this and told us about Richard's new diet tactic. "Well, his ex, really was into her food and started to become a vegan."

Both I and Charlene were left open-mouthed and looking at each other. Charlene closed her mouth to say, "Oh yeah, lots of people are doing that around the flocks in this area. I think Burley has a flock who are pushing veganism, but I could be wrong."

Well, this is something I should think about to make myself more appealing to Richard, at least we'll have lots of good conversation. I looked at Charlene and raised my eyebrows and said, "Well, this is something we could both try and make us more appealing to local rams. What do you think?"

Charlene looked slightly happy and was thinking, which made her look slightly strange, and I suspected that she would say something brilliant about now.

"So, vegans don't eat any meat at all, like no animal stuff, right?"

This is when William burst into the conversation by saying, "Yes! Like nothing at all, basically everything you like!"

I took a gasp, so I won't be able to eat any cakes or cookies. Well, this doesn't seem like living at all.

"Oh dear, Charlene, I don't think we can go to the cookie shop anymore, it's like most of the food we love is taken away from us."

Charlene scorned at me and pushed her wineglass away from her on the table whilst shaking her head.

I felt a sudden urge to carry out this vegan plan thing on my own. I needed to look at it more and explore what is the best way to go about this new way of life style.

If I can do this, I would be in good stead to capturing this Richard and making him mine! This is something that will be difficult, but I reckon I could do this and was looking forward to getting home and opening my laptop to find out more information online. I grabbed my wineglass and slurped away and casually looked down the table at Richard and thought, I wish you knew what I was going to do for you. I slowly stood up and waved my hoof over Steve and William, and air kissed Charlene farewell. I then looked back to see Richard for the final time that night.

Chapter 3

The next morning, I decided to allow myself some hangover time before beginning this vegan research time, mostly because I felt shattered from the previous night's pub dwelling and trotting for more than I had to. Charlene and I have always recognised that getting a taxi back to the farm after three glasses of wine is most preferable, it makes us look classier and established than previous staggering across the country fields and mud pools. I didn't opt for that and prized open my laptop with muddy legs and thought about having a wash and getting clean. Nothing like that happened because I acknowledged the notion that I was still existing in the hangover time so thought it best to lie down first before any high level of research could take place. Thankfully, a bovine thought it best to conduct its morning calls near to where I was. The moos served as a great alarm clock to make me feel alerted and aware.

The laptop awoke, and I did a morning stretch with my arms directly above my head. I rubbed my hoofs together because that's what characters do before any cognitive work, so I thought it best to join that mindset. The beginning start for my internet search was typing the words; HOW TO BE VEGAN. The result was unexpected because there were loads of results, not the three I thought it would be. It would take me forever to look at each result and gain a clearer view of this diet which from what I learnt was the diet of unhappiness. No cakes. No cookies. No doughnuts? How can anyone genuinely eat this way all of the time? I'm amazed the entire vegan flock of Burley haven't rolled over from complete exhaustion. They probably haven't had a laugh from when they started.

Anyway, the farmer must have been on something because I wasn't aware that you could survive without consuming dairy. That was just an animal's need, right? I've had gallons of lattes and I feel fine, in fact, happier for drinking them. Just considering the notion of a hazelnut latte was enough to spur me out of bed and make me grab my bag and put on my shoes to trot to my local coffee house and order a flat hazelnut latte.

When I slurped all of my coffee, I thought it best to stay on track with my vegan learning. As I had spent all of my life living on a farm, there was probably nothing new to teach me. It won't take long to skim through it. I knew the basics already; no meat, dairy or egg. Oh, and had to remember that fish is a meat. Got it. Richard will be immensely impressed with me when I see him next. My thoughts turned on to that scenario for a few minutes, but I managed to whip myself back to this vegan learning thing.

I stumbled upon a video labelled, 'Dairy is Scary' but I instantly retorted the title. All of the female bovines in my farm enjoyed being pregnant and danced themselves to the farm to get rid of their bulging udders. There's nothing scary about that. Dairy wasn't yielding a machete to anyone. Quite calm, watching them queue up to be milked. Definitely not scary, so I rubbished that claim.

My phone started to buzz, and it didn't take me long to believe that Charlene would be calling me, it was after all under ten hours since I last saw her.

'Shirley! I have some gossip regarding the hunky Richard who you drooled over last night in the pub. Well, he is definitely straight AND SINGLE! I did a quick research visit to Burley in order to check if my notes were correct and in fact what we learnt last night was true, things were broken off between him and his girlfriend.'

I tried my best to remain calm and not get too happy as I knew I'd be disrupted in some way if I was too jubilant. After a good 12 seconds, I threw my hoof in the air and cried out, *'WEEEE!'*

My message screen was open for me to lavish praise on Charlene for her farm nosiness, a skill no other could beat. I decided to really get my head around this veganism thing. If Richard is really keen on it, well, so am I. My thoughts circled around when my vegan start date could be and I had plenty of delicious thoughts, one being that I could sneak in a box of doughnuts before I actually start because I thought that would be the easiest dietary path to take for me.

Thankfully, my thoughts were dramatically shaken by actually watching one of the search items on my list I had asked the email gods for earlier in the day. They were all vegan related, so although I had a sneer on my face when I clicked 'play' I was desperate for something to sway my inbuilt doubtfulness about eating this way. If I could do it then Richard would undoubtfully be impressed and ask to marry me. I was certain this would happen, but I actually had to go through with it, the whole no meat thing. There remained a certain aspect of my brain that was adamant that it must be unhealthy to eat this way, after all surely the farmer would have done so already? Or did I actually have to ask him myself? He would probably just tut at me and shake his head like the time I asked for delivery pizzas to be available for all the workers on the farm. I decided not to bug him again.

Charlene arranged her position to be near me and said, "Do you fancy coming for a walk with me? We could assess more guys and chat. Please come, it's boring where I'm standing at the moment and I need some fresh air after spending the night in a pub with only a gay couple who were, in all honesty, obsessed with each other."

I smiled and completely understood what she was chatting about. I loved the guys dearly, but knew she must have felt like a spare wheel when I left last night. She was my partner in female gossips on the farm so said, "Of course! Let's go for a chin wag!"

The Burley farm was going to be on our list of farms to trot around and natter. On the whole, it was boring nattering topics like who would play you in the story of your life and who would be the heartthrob?

Charlene was most amused by this topic and giggled throughout the five minutes of us bleating away. At one point,

I even put my arm around her for a friendly cuddle. That was an action I've been on the receiving end of a few times, but today I completely understood it.

"So, then, Shirley, have you drawn up an eating plan going forward? I can help you if you like, let's start tomorrow?"

How my mood was shattered by Charlene's speaking moments. I went from happy joy that was shared with my best mate, to cannon ball hitting my stomach. It was an immediate sense of panic as I knew Charlene was right. Like a plaster stuck over skin, the best way to get rid of it was to quickly whip it off. I wouldn't be surprised if Charlene hadn't made an eating plan for me herself.

"I've made a vegan eating plan for you myself!"

My smile needed to fade after hearing that. Was she trying to be mean? She knew we both hated the idea of veganism. She loved eating doughnuts just the same as me. I thought she should be brought down with me on this eating plan. It surprised me even more when she said, "You will join me in this vegan thing, yeah?"

I imagined her to instantly let out a couple of swear words and an enormous 'NO' but she didn't, most worryingly she had her thinking face on. It would only take a few seconds before I heard her answer. Those were the most worrisome seconds of my life, I knew if she joined my vegan attempt then that would be it; no scoffing doughnuts before I start. I looked up at her to receive an answer despite me half knowing what it would be.

"Well, actually, Shirley after what was said about the diet last night, I looked into it and realised it's a good thing. Hell, yeah, I'll join you!"

That cannon ball that hit me earlier came back to hit me again. If I start this then Charlene will make absolutely sure I was following the diet correctly. Any mishap I do will be recorded and acknowledged by Charlene herself. In some ways, she likes picking up on my failures only to inflame her own self confidence. Quite pathetic, I believe. Well, my pre-diet planning has gone up in flames. Surely, I wouldn't be able to scoff my face off at a patisserie now if we're donning the vegan caps tomorrow. Or will it?

"So, Charlene, you know how we're starting veganism tomorrow right? Don't suppose you fancy eating a bucket of doughnuts tonight?"

Charlene carried on in the same tone as I had.

"Yes! Absolutely, we can definitely be vegan once the clock strikes 12!"

I was outstandingly grateful we both shared the same thought regarding the non-vegan treat before slavishly abiding by the vegan rules.

"Okay, Charl, let's go and feast ourselves silly!"

After saying that, I could sense Charlene looking elsewhere. I nipped over to her eyeline and instantly saw where she was looking. Richard and William were both talking with each other. They were too far away to distinguish what they were talking about, but I felt like a student in a classroom breaking away from a lesson. I grabbed Charlene's arm and shouted, "Come on, it's almost sunset! We're vegans tomorrow!"

Chapter 4

The bakery we chose for our last time to be deviant, before the vegan axe came down, was tucked away in the village near our farm. I was impressed by how much my predictive doughnut thoughts turned out to be true, the entire bucket was grabbed and yanked to where we decided to sit. We took it in turns to grasp each doughnut and smash it into our open mouths, leaving sugar trails all over our table. Charlene even thought she'd make the evidence go away by swiping our table. I didn't let her know the bakery employees would come and clean each table by the end of the night. I knew this because of a past visit here, I didn't buy a bucket of doughnuts then, but a sensible amount for my stomach – just two doughnuts to share between me and my ex, Claude. The thought of him still marginally brought up feelings of annoyance. Maybe, I should have delayed thinking such thoughts by another two years.

Charlene did a loud swallow, then began to speak, "I wonder what William and Richard spoke about when we saw them earlier."

I prepared my mouth ready to speak by dusting off the sugar from my lips then said, "I don't know, maybe football? Richard apparently likes that."

We needed to time when we spoke to each other to be consistent with when we ate, otherwise the questions would be left with a blank reply. When there was a pause, I gave the suggestion of us going back to the farm when the bucket was empty. Charlene gave an upbeat sound, and I took the last doughnut.

"So okay, Shirl, I have created what we should eat tomorrow."

A vicious snarl left my lips and shouted, "Why have you done that?"

I was still anti anything vegan until the next day. In fact, I believed it was just wrong and rude to mention anything vegan to my face. I needed to display my feelings regarding this.

Charlene wasn't deterred and offered a peace deal regarding tomorrow's food, "How about you come to mine for breakfast and we could eat some oats with blueberries?"

Instantly snapping again, I stood and shouted, "PAH!"

A semblance of pity was held by myself for Charlene, she was probably doing her best to make me happy but unfortunately, I wasn't in the mood, especially after my doughnut gut bloating. No not yet, maybe tomorrow. And that was a maybe.

As we lugubriously trotted, we passed the sports fields on our left. There were a group of people standing at the corner of the marked ground. I needed to stop and perform a move that many actors follow by raising a palm above the eyeline to cut out the sun rays. When I looked at the group of people, who were around ten in number, I realised they were clad in plastic sportswear. There was one member of the sport clan who was marching away by himself. Or could it be herself? It was difficult to tell from this distance. Whatever the gender of them, they were marching towards us.

I cut back to what Charlene was talking to herself about.

"It's 500 grams of plain flour, then 150 grams of sugar then olive oil. I can't remember the technical cooking amounts, but I can look that up when I get back to the farm. So, then I put it all in a bowl and mix it all up! I'll probably do it when we get back because then we just have to fire up the stove, so we can pour out the pancake mix for tomorrow morning!"

Charlene the chef, was very excited about doing this. I was more excited about getting back to the barn so I could laze in front of the television to watch a box set. Or two, depending on what's on offer.

When I looked up, I could tell 100% the lone person who broke away from the group was male. Charlene who stood to my left suddenly gasped and was left ash faced and wide mouthed.

I had no idea what the cause of this was, although the doughnut gut stuffing probably had something to do with it. She raised her hoof in the direction of the male coming towards us and near whispered to me, "That is Richard! We haven't any time before he reaches us!"

I shushed her to be quiet and worked on my own internal status. I was far away from panicking if Richard was choosing to speak with me, but I needed to come up with something to talk about. And oh my goodness, he was coming over to me and oh my goodness the doughnuts I'm digesting suddenly wanted to do an air somersault in my stomach. The globules of sweat I had suddenly amassed needed to be wiped away from my head and I thought it best to use my right wrist to push the liquid away from my head. And wow, he's a fast walker. In less than a bovine roll he was stood directly opposite us with a smile.

Despite desperately wanting to stand and look at him smiling, producing a blaze of white teeth, I thought it best to say something so offered a "hi".

Without thinking much, I recoiled and spent the next 30 seconds looking at his glorious face. I felt an overwhelming sense of pride he honoured us with his time and walking across the sport's field to converse with us. I felt so much pride that even the digesting doughnuts wanted to join it and somersaulted three times. My belly gurgle felt loud enough, even the caretaker of the sports ground could probably hear. Richard just looked up and into my eyes and offered a caring small smile.

This was something my digesting doughnuts really enjoyed and went for a five-time flip. My annoyance at my own tummy grew exponentially with each belly flop. Did my tummy not realise the gentle ram who I was endlessly staring at the other night stood right opposite me? I gave myself a weak happy sigh and then refocused on what to do and say.

This was going to be a hard task during my bout of doughnut dancing occurring in my tummy, but I still wanted to try, he could be wanting a date with me. Maybe that was what he was talking with William about? That would make the most sense and if it were true then I should try my best to graciously receive such an offer for a date. Should I courtesy? Or would that be odd? I suddenly gathered that Charlene was nodding in my peripheral vision but what was she nodding about?

Richard increased his impressive factor by opting to speak about a topic I had previously positioned in my rhetoric to chat about for conversations with William in order to ensure a pub visit was established. Seeing the gorgeous Richard standing in front of us, it seemed pointless that used too much brain juice.

With that thought, my stomach released a gargantuan roar and I felt uneasy. I then prayed for my gut not to do what I feared it would. It did try a little, but I managed to keep down a small burp both physically and audibly. I thought. Richard thought it best to offer a question at this time.

"What are you two ewes doing today?"

It was at this specific moment my gut worked its hardest to unload its holdings and pushed them up to the nearest available exit also known as my mouth. I couldn't prevent the massive splurge from happening and guessing was pushed backwards in order to see the acidic pool. Richard was standing cross armed with one finger on his chin.

Oh jeez, talk about creating an opinion. I couldn't see any come back from this, so I didn't even want to say anything at all, especially as I felt droplets of vomit still on my chin. I was quite satisfied to leave any talking with Charlene, so I kept concentrating on breathing with my ears open.

"Well, today we were going to head back to our barn to rest, and in Shirley's position, recuperate!"

Richard's eyebrows raised, and he nodded slowly.

"I was actually coming over to see if Shirley wanted to go for a drink but by seeing that, I'm guessing that's a no!"

In my mind, I was screaming phrases like, 'YES' but my mouth and head remained in the same position. Thankfully, my best friend came to my rescue. I really should improve my reference of her from 'acquaintance' up to 'best friend'. Especially answering Richard like this, "Shirley would very much like to have a drink with you, she has told me specifically about you. Obviously not now. Tomorrow will be a better day as we're both adopting a vegan diet." Enough I had my head close to the ground I could tell Charlene was emitting the feeling of smugness.

I pushed myself up on my four feet and daren't give Richard a look. He was still devilishly good looking but held a face I wasn't aware of. He looked as though he was in some sort of pain with wrinkled brows and wide eyes staring at me. I wasn't sure if I appreciated that look to be honest. I much preferred his smiling face.

"Well, that's great, maybe we can be in contact in a few weekends time. It takes a couple of weeks to get a sense of normality after starting veganism. Trust me, I've only just started myself! Right, best go, I think you need to tend to this patient." With that, Richard bowed towards me.

After raising my head, a small amount of vomit dribbled out of my mouth.

Thankfully, I didn't have to worry about causing any more embarrassment as I heard Richard stomp away with his voice's volume slowly reducing.

Chapter 5

My legs felt worn out like I had just finished a long running race. Waking up brought new acknowledgements of different parts of my body hurting. I couldn't remember what kind of drinks I drank last night, but I did know they must have been strong as my chest felt weakened. I only just realised it was Charlene, standing by the front door. How odd she was to be standing there, I would have expected a text to announce that she was coming over. I didn't see her much after leaving Fawcett fields, have been eating lots of doughnuts. And ahoy, a memory just smacked me round the head; I was sick all over the gravel car park. I can remember that as clear as day. There was a viewer, standing at the gravel's edge and oh yes, that was Richard. He was a sheep who I couldn't possibly woo over with my charm anymore, even I could tell as it was truly hideous vomiting. Charlene did her best to calm me and encourage interactions with him going forward, he said things that were 'caring'.

Why wasn't Charlene feeling this pain? She did after all consume the same number of doughnuts as I did, why didn't she throw up too? That would have made it nicer for me and not solemnly dealing with the vomit gate all by myself. It was after all rude not to vomit next to me. That wouldn't be as dismaying of me by Richard.

On the stumble back to the barn, Charlene was keen to let me know that Richard really did offer caring words and still wants to go out with me. He thought us going vegan was a noble thing to do but he did say it takes a few weeks for the gut to acclimatise. He said that he knew all that because he went vegan. Something to talk with him about eh, Shirl?

Suddenly, my memory cleared its self-up regarding, getting back to the barn. The TV show I pleaded with Charlene to watch as well as pulling the duvet up to my head, I must have fallen asleep at that point.

If Richard was very keen on this vegan malarkey then why haven't I been fed? I best ask the chef.

"Charlene? Where's my breakfast? I thought you told me about ingredients yesterday? I'm starting to get hungry now."

There was rustling by the duvet cover on the other side of the room, I squinted to make the image clearer for me. A blonde headed bobble squeezed out between the wall and the duvet cover, it was Charlene who groaned and said, "It's in the kitchen, start up the oven and we can make the pancakes from there."

I didn't appreciate her collapsing under the duvet again. We needed to get going to get the vegan wheels going. Maybe I should give her a prod to enlighten her? The loud ugly snoring dissuaded me from doing such an action, so I felt a rush of feminine power and went to the kitchen to do this chef thing all by myself. If I could get the bowl with the ingredients already prepared, it could become okay. Now, I needed to switch on the oven, how would I do that? I riffled through my memory bank to find a sense of help. Yes, I remember being in the kitchen one time and Claude jumped in to save the hungry situation we were in. Yes, he moved round the back of the cooker and switched something on. I should perform the same actions.

Once I woke up the cooker by making it give an almighty growl, I saw a figure walk in, giving themselves a stretch. It was my sleeping friend, Charlene, awake and rubbing her eyes to fully adjust to the new day. Thought it best to fully wake her up by saying, "Morning, Charlene! Are you surprised I have done this much so far?"

The pancakes boomed in size from the near moment we placed the beige thick droplets on the sizzling saucepan. I didn't want to admit it, but the smell that occurred was wonderful, it made me feel more confident in joining this vegan gang.

This is good! Thank you for starting this up, I was proper dozing. I blame the doughnuts for knocking me for six.

I immediately relaxed back a retort about her not spewing her guts out like me. A cutting remark after we were having a good time scoffing our faces like how we were with the doughnuts. I thought it best to put forward a question relating to me dramatically vomiting again. Thankfully, Charlene delivered the news with a smile.

"It's all right, Shirley, you can eat however much vegan food you like and not throw up!" I considered making another batch of pancakes but then settled on eating the remaining blueberries instead of doing any chef work.

I was dumbfounded by the fact I could eat everything on the vegan diet and not puke out dinner. Charlene must have been wrong when she said that, surely my stomach would hastily remove food items if it got too crowded? I needed to press Charlene on this matter, as I was looking after her phone when she went out. I was alerted to it ringing and not breaking any rules by looking, so I gauged the caller.

Who was Barry? It didn't alert any of my recognitions as to who he was. That's if it's a ram. There's been an awful lot of cat fishing around this area, sheep who lie about their appearance online. Ewes pretending to be rams and vice versa. I will have to wait until I can grab Charlene to give me an explanation about who this 'Barry' was and why he would call her. After about three hours, Charlene showed her face. I jumped at the chance to quiz her as soon as I could.

"So, who's this Barry? Why was he calling you?"

I have been told I should lessen the demanding nature of how my questions were delivered but for this question, I really wanted to know. I believed my tactful nature on this occasion was displayed because I didn't use any force.

Charlene noticed my presence and gave a small nod. I didn't know how to comprehend, did I do something right? Something I wasn't aware of? I thought it best to offer a face that just screamed 'ANSWER ME'. I gave her approximately one minute to answer me. When she passed that timing guide, I thought it best to speak.

"So yes, I'm sorry for seeing your home screen when it rang but the contact name came up when your phone rang, I had to look in case it was an urgent call you needed to know straight away and not deviant to another farm like you usually do."

I thought it was time to raise my eyebrows to add to the sense of need for an answer I was emitting. This tactic didn't work so I would have to revert to inventing a reason with regard to this 'Barry'. Could he be one of Charlene's cousin's? Or maybe he was her secret lover or maybe a bespoke photographer? Or maybe he was a gossip scout that feeds her new information that she could feed back to me?

These predictions seemed perfectly true and believable, I didn't have a problem in offering Charlene the option to answer.

It was a disappointment to hear that they were all false. She didn't have to enter a loud case after each refusal. Her cackling after I asked about Barry being her lover felt a bit mean.

"I think you'll really like him, he's previously asked me about you, Shirley! It's only recently since I've been in contact with him. By us going vegan, I thought it best to have a nutritionist to guide us."

I didn't predict that. I thought it best to offer my thoughts on the matter.

"Well done, Charlene but couldn't you get all of the nutritional information and recipes from the internet?"

A deep sigh was had by her and I think Charlene was thinking about speaking. I wasn't keen to take opinion on this matter, mostly because I didn't spend enough time on vegan research. I will probably be able to pick up on whatever science is presented to me regarding eating.

"There are plenty of sites that give information about what to eat on a vegan diet. In fact, Barry gave me an acronym to remember what should be included in meals on a vegan diet."

I was slightly confused as to what an acronym could be, surely it's to do with not eating any meat, dairy or eggs. I don't understand what more of an acronym could be.

"I think Barry gave me the best acronym, it's Gbombs!"

I just looked at Charlene continuously. Did she expect me to understand what she was going on about? She mentioned the word 'bombs'. I thought vegan was a diet that was peaceful and serene not argumentative bearing weapons. Not using bombs.

"So, what does Gbombs mean? And how do we eat a bomb?"

This made Charlene burst with excitement leaning across to me.

"Well, G stands for greens, B stands for beans, O stands for onions, M stands for mushrooms, B stands for berries and S stands for seeds."

"Wow, Charlene! That's impressive. How long did it take to learn that? It sounds very cool, although I was hoping the M would stand for meat."

Charlene instantly tutted at me, but I still didn't understand what I did wrong. I genuinely didn't feel meat should be completely off of the eating list. The only thing making me comply is meeting and talking with Richard. If I even sniffed at a slice of meat, Richard would probably be able to tell.

Chapter 6

Considering William's reason for calling, I was drawing blanks. He wasn't sexually attracted to her as he has a boyfriend and probably thought of Charlene as an immediate no-go area. Not a thought about her romantically happened, the best assumption I could gather is that William had some dramatic gossip to share with Charlene. That must have been it because I couldn't contemplate anything else. The sound of her trotting got me excited to find exactly what the topic was on the phone last night.

"Shirley? Are you in? I've got something important to tell you. It's about Richard."

Those sounds made me jump to attention, why did Richard have to be brought into this? Couldn't he have just remained on the side-lines?

"So, William told me about how deadly serious he was about taking you out on a date. Apparently, he's had a crush on you for a while."

This news just met an uninterested face. I was not aware of Richard having a crush on me, in fact he could have learnt how to cartwheel and display it on the hills and I still wouldn't be interested. Not even a spark occurred after that Richard news. From what I honestly thought of him, he couldn't do anything to impress me. Maybe in another life we could be married and swimming in children

Him, looking down on me when I puked multiple times after eating lots of doughnuts was enough to erase him from my memory. He could never think of me as an attractive ewe, so I might as well block the entrance of romantic thoughts involving Richard. I can't believe eating vegan would make him swoon over me, what a turd I was. A blip of sorrow flew over me then.

"Richard is still really keen to meet you! Even after you threw up most of your interior in the Fawcett carpark. William was being honest when he told me, and I believe him totally. He told me to mention that fact to you, so I have!"

I didn't appreciate her trying to be honest, with a smile after speaking so I shrugged it off. If Richard was truly honest in liking me then he could have made it obvious to me. A tiny part of my ego blames me for puking up to a large extent. We needed to eat in a non-vegan meal because we were determined to go vegan the next day, if I didn't know of vegan Richard, I wouldn't have stuffed my stomach with so many doughnuts, so with this in consideration Richard was to blame for the massive spell of vomit. I hated him.

I enquired as to what we were going to eat. The vegan menu was just insane madness to me. Couldn't we just get a takeaway pizza? I didn't care about it being dairy and not vegan. I really thought it was a stupid idea. *Yeah, there are lots of articles really selling it up and all but how can we boring unexcited sheep really think we could do it? Everyone else on the farm were happy to chomp down on burgers and sausages. Maybe I should join them, I would be happier with that menu! I just needed to make that selection to Charlene. It does after all, lessen her cooking time, she stubbornly takes on herself to do. Feeling selfish, I have offered to help but after ten times being told to "Just stand there, out of the way".*

I love it when a plan formulates, so my new plan of action was to trot down to the village high street and get my hooves on a fast-food takeaway meal. My saliva glands in my mouth were getting excited just thinking about it.

I packed my bag to escape this farm and go on my sneaky high street mission but unfortunately, Charlene thought it best to speak.

"Where are you going? Don't you want to get some food?"

The tut just jumped from my mouth. My honest side whizzed in to give an answer.

"I'm going to the high street actually to visit Ronald's. We've been there before. Do you remember?"

I gave a holy smile to join with my honest side. Charlene would understand, we've been in that eating establishment many times before. She didn't need to look possessed but the loud shrill of her shouting and holding the same note became eerie and shocking.

Despite me putting my hoof over hers, she still seemed mightily annoyed and judging by her left water logged eyeball, looked upset too.

"Why do you have to ruin everything, Shirley? Why can't you just stay with a plan of action with anything in your life? Is that why you dumped Claude?"

It was my turn to get annoyed and shout now.

"I didn't dump Claude, Char, he dumped me. Thank you for reminding me of that fact, Char. The worst moment of my life. Thanks for the reminder."

Without meaning to, a large globule of tear ran down my left cheek. Those two seconds would have won an Oscar. Charlene grabbed my arm and pulled me up to meet her marching to the door. I needed to check where she was going. I didn't want to be pulled into something that was not desirable. She's done that before when she pushed me into studio for me to de-robe and be a model of a live drawing class. I hope she wasn't pulling me for that.

"Come on, let's go to the place you are so desperate to go to. Is it a burger you want?"

Charlene appeared to me as cocky and mean. I hadn't done anything to provoke her. Yes, I told her in no uncertain terms that I wanted to stop being a veganista by going to the Ronald's but surely, she shouldn't have been so rude by yanking me out of the barn with her?

We reached the ordering counter and I realised Charlene was looking at me with slightly raised eyebrow in a look that dared me to order.

In loud clear language and tone, I gave my order.

"Double burger with cheese please."

The burger maid quickly chirped a 'thank you' and spun around to quickly gain the order from the beef rack.

I flashed a smile and scooped up my order in my hooves and beckoned Charlene to leave the restaurant with me. She followed me to the nearest park bench, and we perched as I opened my goods. I was only two mouthfuls in when I thought it was important to ask a question much needed to be answered, "Was it always this salty before? We used to eat loads of these every day."

After saying that, I hocked up a heavy spit ball, I chucked on the pavement. It was absolutely disgusting. All I wanted was a nice warm soup to hopefully get rid of the taste of salt.

"Come on, Shirley, let's go back to the barn. There's a film you said you wanted to see the other week. It's on the telly so we could watch that?"

I'm so thankful to my new best friend, she has fulfilled her best friend daily quota by saying those words. The tacky ringing from her phone ruined my peaceful moment to myself. This could be a fun time to eavesdrop, so I moved closer to her. It was definitely a male as I could hear his baritone coming out of the phone. My ears pricked up with excitement; for my whole life, I have been interested in rams. I don't see why I should stop now.

Charlene gave me a glance and she let out a giggle. She looked at me and said, "And you speak with Shirley for a bit please, Barry? She didn't realise how salty burgers are."

Did I really need to feel like a child with you saying a thing like that? I deducted ten new best friend points from her. She tried her best to look caring but failed by the time I swiped her phone from her. I wanted to retain my impeccable new best friend record by gently holding the phone to my ear and politely saying, "Hello?"

Barry took a moment before he made an answer, "Hi, Shirley, Charlene has told me you have dropped out of veganism?"

Oh drat. I will need to answer that question. Of course, I have tried life outside the VG plates Charlene has probably spoken on numerous occasions about what we're doing in the vegan world so it will be frankly annoying to answer you.

"Yes, I have, Barry."

Using the first name was a good trick to use as it made me feel superior and Barry a lesser sheep in the diarchy of us talking. He hummed and began to speak again.

"That's great! Well done to you for giving it a go. Charlene tells me you found the burger you bought was salty?"

Again, a stupid thing to ask me. I was perfectly aware of what Charlene said to him on the phone before she passed the handset to me. I spent a moment for him to stew on his question but thought it best to say something as I could be on speakerphone. My answer was droll and unsurprising. Using a monotone could be used to let him know I was aware of his silly questions. I really hoped Charlene was listening.

"Yes, that's right. The burger was really salty."

There was complete silence from his end, so I thought it best to have fun. The only audience member was me during the conversation.

"It made me feel really poor, Barry! How could it be so mean? Help me, Barry!"

I chuckled to myself in my head. I was waiting for his ball to be served.

"Well, Shirley, you're not alone in saying this, when you're a vegan your taste buds expand to taste the good flavours of everything you eat. By eating something that has salt in it just sends a clear message to the brain not to eat it."

So that was a victory for Barry.

Chapter 7

On the morning when I rose to assess another day, I noticed it was crisp innocent morning, with a placement of coldness without being cold. There were no signs of ice on the pathways, but I wouldn't have been surprised if my eyes were to suddenly find a pocket of ice somewhere on the path. From where I stood outside of the barn, I experienced a whoosh of smell coming from the cow barn. For whatever reason, I had never smelled the cow's manure with this potency before. The farmer might not have had time to clean their barn fully, I'm certain he would do so today if he had time. Now my tummy grumbled so I singularly thought about feeding myself. With a rush of power and knowledge that I had around an hour before my grazing duty was to start, I strutted to open the food cupboard to see what food options were available to me.

After Barry's phone call last night, I decided to have a vegan diet. This decision was made by me and not forced on me by the farmer, Charlene, or any other sheep. It was especially not forced by the sheep at Burley Farm, although they did look magnificent by their vegan diet. This new attacking of the vegan diet was down to me and only me Shirley S Sheep. What could I see here amongst the stash of the food cupboard?

I plucked down a carton of cereal for me to sit and look at the ingredients list. This was something I never did, normally as I relied upon other sheep more specifically, Charlene who outlined what I could and couldn't eat every day. I saluted the vegan gods as they had placed their logo on the back of the cereal box to prevent me from wasting my time trawling through each to check if it is an animal product. Thankfully, I couldn't find anything, so I felt the most jubilant feeling like the feeling I had realising pasta is an innocent food dish that could, forever more be eaten without any sense of guilt. I nodded to the logo to give a sign of agreement with it. A nod. That is if no sneaky eggs had niggled in to the ingredients list.

After eating my breakfast and placing my bowl on the side of the kitchen counter, I decided to put my war paint, aka make-up, on before work began. To think of anything more serious was being rude to any delicate make up movements I was to make to my face. Especially if I worked on my eyeline. I didn't want to create black sploshes. Even Burley ewes didn't have those.

With the start of the grazing due to happen in twenty minutes, I was surprised Charlene hadn't text me. Normally, I would receive a daily rundown of the day's news which were mostly gossip related and useless, but I didn't have to wait long for a call.

"Shirley? Are you ready to go to work?"

There have been times when I needed more boudoir prep before sitting and listening to a news rundown before work. So, I told her I was ready.

"So, the Burley farm are all a whizz, when I left you last night, I found out exactly what was causing this. Your ram, Richard, was causing a stir in the ewe delegation of the farm."

I became overwhelmingly agitated by her using the term 'your ram' because Richard was in no way associated with me. To assume he was, was just lazy in speaking terms. I would have much preferred something like, 'That sheep who you really fancy' as a term which she could have used in alternative meaning. I needed to instantly quieten her for me to set her right.

"Charlene! Please don't call Richard my ram because if that was true, wouldn't I be rocking a diamond on my left hoof? Don't ever say that again."

I needed to claim out one possibility that could occur however, if Richard did propose to me then I wouldn't be offended by the term she said to me. I'd be perfectly happy from the next moment when I said 'yes' to him but unfortunately, I've turned away from thinking about him so will not go anywhere near the path of wishing what could happen. I've learnt my lesson after thinking penguins could genuinely fly and asking everyone around the farm to come with me on a safari around the artic to watch the penguins fly to migrate. The farm just snootily laughed at me and pulled faces, imploring me to continue talking, this was something where I learnt about thinking about future opportunities. Richard was one of those.

"Okay, okay! I won't mention something like that again. The Burley farm was however, buzzing with excitement that Richard and his girlfriend had announced their marriage. I wouldn't be sad about it, Shirl, they've been on the rocks for a while before he joined us for dinner. It's not as bigger news the Burley clan make it out to be."

I offered Charlene a rewarding smile, despite being unseen on the phone, to thank her for the news and trotted off to the farm for work.

The smell of the grass was quite rewarding as it masked the stench of the cow mess I woke up to. With the fields being mown and the dainty aroma wafting over the field, I felt at least happier where I chose to conduct my grazing. My darling friend, Charlene, chose to graze near me and disrupt my morning's meditation. Hopefully, she would be mute unless something was communicated to me of vital importance.

"Shirley, do you fancy going up to the high street sometime? Barry's told me about this new rice bar that is apparently excellent and has received multiple awards. Rice is vegan you know."

I completely didn't even consider the little white flakes that were rice when I ran through what foods were on the vegan list, probably because of the exquisite happiness of pasta being truly vegan.

Yes, of course, rice was, they were mini clumps of pasta wannabes weren't they? I should remain calm when answering because I didn't want Charlene to think I didn't know rice was vegan. I didn't actually know that, but I didn't want the same type of reaction of when I wanted to see the penguin flight migration. To my utter shame, I found out that penguins don't fly. They swim a lot.

"Yes, that would be good, Char, let's go next week? I've got lots of that batch of stir fry using those Gbombs that Barry told us about. We will not starve until then!"

Charlene looked excited and nodded to then reveal a cheeky looking smile.

"I knew you'd say yes to the invitation! I'll pass over some dried noodles that I picked up on my shopping trip recently, you could call it payback for the glasses of wine we've glugged through over the time we turned vegan."

A sheep who was a stranger to us, barged past the other sheep who were in the way of him getting to us for some reason. When he stood mostly by Charlene, when he started to yelp out these brutal set of words.

"When will you shut up about vegan stuff? I understand it's your diet, but can you give it a rest and not say anything more about it around here? I eat plenty of meat every day and I'm still alive, so I don't need to think about changing my diet."

Charlene surprised me as she didn't break her smile for the entire stranger's talking. Pretty impressive, after all the vegan insults. She quickly sighed and prepared to speak. Something she has always shied away from regarding talking to a stranger.

"Thanks for your input stranger, even though I'm not a doctor, I can swear to you that eating meat each morning will probably kill you."

The stranger sighed at her and let out a chuckle. These actions didn't halt Charlene from speaking.

"You do know that every mouthful you ingest leaves a trail of plaque? The more you eat meat, the more arteries gain lots of plaques. I'm surprised you haven't had a heart attack already."

To our surprise, the stranger began to gentle stomp his hooves and looked squarely at Char. I hoped he wasn't going to unleash anymore harsh words because that would have upset her innocence. I've already used up all the tissues I had for her crying and sniffing up snot.

"Do you know me or what happened to me last month? I was rushed to the vets because they thought I had a heart attack. Are you telling me I shouldn't eat any meat at all? Wow, way to ruin my day sweetheart, but because you're nice and seem knowledgeable about these things I'll give it a go. You know, veganism. If you think it's best."

Nothing could have stopped Charlene from bounding up to him that she needed to get a hand out regarding a six-day vegan challenge. Apparently, it really works to gain lifelong vegans, something she was keen to point out when she read the internet page.

"No more meat for you, I'd say and appreciate the fruit and veg when you can." Feeling the need to offer options to him, I gave him a simple offer.

"Pasta is vegan you know, not the creamy type but the dry sort, you know?"

The stranger smiled broadly and gave Charlene a cheeky wink. Presumable, Barry taught Charlene everything she needed to know about veganism and its health benefits. Something I bet she couldn't wait to get off her chest to someone new. Having a stranger against her, in certain terms, was like winning the lottery for her.

"That's good to know, I'll let you know how I get on doctor!"

When I arrived home, I felt satisfied. We could have saved a life.

Chapter 8

After my morning start up rituals, like eating breakfast and smiling smugly to myself, I was entering another day in the world being vegan. This was a genuine skill I could be proud of. I thought about other tasks I could achieve as Charlene and I obviously saved the life of a stranger yesterday. Maybe I could convince more strangers to stop eating meat? I'm sure Charlene could help me with this. Right now, I needed to concentrate on my morning rituals.

My phone rang just as I opened my make-up bag to begin the morning ritual of applying coloured creams to my face as well as powders to my eyelids, so I answered the phone call. It didn't surprise me; it was Charlene wanting a chat.

"So, I have news! The ferry came in and docked from the continent and new sheep have come to the area and are looking for jobs!"

I pulled my phone away from my ear so I could make a big shrug and say "who cares?" but I obediently listened to her saying more as it just might be relevant to me.

"Yes, the population of the area will increase and there's one sheep who has arrived and been trotting around here who's relevant to you."

My ears pricked up to hear more. She needs to divulge me more regarding how it is relevant to only me. Most of my life has been living amongst the herd so it's welcomed to hear something specifically for me. This will be fun to learn about. I hope she doesn't say something completely meaningless and notion it about it being just for me.

"So, I watched when the new sheep disembarked from the ferry and one face stood out to me. Shirley, I think it was

Claude, your ex. I couldn't be deadly sure if it was him because I was quite far away, but he certainly looked familiar. You ready for work? I'm off now."

What a bomb relevant to me, to deal with. I'll give her praise as the news was specific to me. So, I'll welcome that. Charlene hasn't actually been my best friend for that long, probably three years at best count so I'd be surprised to hear if she's actually met him. It was probably best to think Claude wasn't here and back home in France. Yes, that would be good as after being dumped and calling off our wedding he retreated to his family home and switched off his phone. The nastiness of it still affects me today.

When I meandered around the sheep field, I couldn't stop my thoughts and feelings to occur. However, I repeated the mantra 'he is a pointless turd'. And if a Claude thought flickered in my brain, I would say the mantra ten times more. I will not waste my precious time on this planet thinking about worthless beings like Claude.

My grazing position is brilliant to aptly offer me entertainment with a good view of the high street. When a morning's work is done, I can allow my gaze to wander to find more entertainment at the high street. Sometimes, the street is full of floats with carnival sounds which raise my mood. Although, sometimes, the street might have a single individual spitting or throwing up. Those were the best moments. For now, I just had the unexciting work to do without thinking about Claude. It would be good to have someone like my new best friend to chat to in order to move my thought tracks away from Claude.

"Hey, Shirley, what's happening? Been up to much today, after I told you about Claude arriving to this area?"

That was an idiotic thing to ask because I haven't moved from the same spot where we both usually stand and do nothing exciting. The Claude news was marginally interesting, but I don't really care about that. Much because he dumped me. I mean, I hope he is well and all that but to me he is a pointless turd.

"How do you feel about going to that noodle bar that we spoke about at lunchtime?"

My lunch and dinner plans, using Barry's Gbombs, were obviously ignored but I did feel hungry. I offered my acceptance.

Charlene did mention my earlier plans to eat the prepared and gave a forced smile, then grabbed my arm like she forced me to eat a burger. We jollied down the pathways, then paused as we entered the fluorescent signed bar. Why were there lots of people? Did Charlene organise this? I wouldn't put it past her.

"Whose birthday is it Charlene? Why is it so crowded?"

"I'm not sure, maybe it's a known vegan noodle bar and sheep just flock to it?"

I looked across at the herd, it had none of my farm attending. There were, however, lots of sheep from Burley farm. Otherwise, known as vegan town.

A handful of sheep, next stepped through the doors, they were sheep who I recognised. Richard, who has been labelled mine but is not, William who if I can remember is his best mate and a female. She was presumably his girlfriend. I looked at Charlene who probably saw everything I saw regarding the trio's entrance.

Charlene moved to me before we would gain a place to eat and said quietly with her head looking down, "That ewe is called Chloe, she's Richard's new girlfriend. I didn't realise Richard would come here!"

That was a bet I would take. Charlene knows everything about everyone. Oh, hold up, this Chloe was packing up her bag and stood to leave. She shot Richard a view and then shrugged.

My eyes didn't deceive me as I saw Chloe trot in to the fast food place where I went to eat that salty burger. I had a little chuckle to myself as her actions demonstrated she wasn't a super keen vegan because she was dating one; Richard, who was.

"Chloe's gone in to that fast-food place Ronald's, that leaves the door open wide for me who has been a justified vegan for two weeks now."

I looked to gain a nod regarding how long I've been a vegan from Charlene. She was more consumed regarding her nails than me.

Chapter 9

After finding out that bombshell of Charlene dating a sheep who is famous, my morning rituals were much more enticing to undertake. I left my duvet in much gusto with a smile to make my cornflakes, which were genuine vegan as it had the official stamp of vegan on its box, to then receive the daily phone natter with Charlene. A call without the large report with the details of how the couple met, best features, when she will say she loves him. On that last point, Charlene scoffed at me and said, "Whenever it feels right."

On the commute to work, I let out a skip when I was almost at the field, something I hadn't done for many years as I'm fully aware that I'm not a lamb anymore. It felt fun to mimic though, and in my mind, I scheduled to do again many times going forward. The action must be like a sporting habit, so must burn lots of calories, so will work on shedding the pounds of fat I had built up.

I spotted Charlene, walking up the hill, I beckoned her over to me.

"CHARLENE!"

She must have appreciated that. She was, after all, my new best friend so would appreciate being wanted by me.

When she settled in her grazing position, it opened my speech cue.

"I'm still amazed at just the level of attention Barry had last night, like proper A list. You certainly got a good catch with him."

As there was silence after saying that, I quickly offered a follow up question.

"How are you feeling? I didn't receive a call from you this morning, which is unusual, but all right."

I gave a fake laugh to ease her into giving an answer.

"I feel fine, just a bit tired after staying awake with Barry last night until midnight. I followed Burley's trend of not wearing any make-up at all, did you realise?"

Of course, I realised. A splash of clear lip gloss wouldn't have gone a miss if I did that.

"Of course, I realised, your face looks really young and fresh. Do you two want to go out for a drink tonight?"

I've never seen Charlene wince as she did. Thankfully, she gave an answer to accustom that expression.

"Umm, I don't think so. Barry gets recognised wherever he goes. Do you want to come around to mine?"

This was a decent plan from Charlene because where I live is just next door so wouldn't be a tiresome commute like getting into somewhere busy like a city or anything. Yes, hopefully, the couple won't be embarrassing, like groom each other using their mouths. Preparation in that scenario occurring was already inked up to prepare; the evil death stare, mammoth tut, and strong head shakes were willing to be unleashed should the motions arise.

Charlene gave a sneaky giggle to that and blew a kiss after meeting her lips with her hoof.

The grazing work, the farmer had outlined for us to do, needed to be done, so we trotted off to our field areas to get munching, the sooner we could start, the sooner we could finish was the motto I've lived my entire life on.

There was a huddle of sheep chatting and laughing about something, but I didn't want to break my work rule about working to finish as it would mean breaking away from what I've been doing and going down there, a good two minutes' worth of grass shearing would be lost in doing so. Without a warning, Charlene swooped into my field of vision and squeaked at me to hurry up and join her to investigate what was going on with the crowd at the far end. I agreed so Charlene performed her much used manoeuvres of grabbing my arm and yanking me in the direction she wanted to go.

The sound volume soared, the closer we arrived in the middle of the flock. My ears twanged when I heard ewes say things like, "I love his accent! He sounds so sexy!"

They were the thoughts I had with my ex, but those sexy sounds turned into him leaving me at the altar. As it was coming to almost five mutes away from my grazing area I turned to return.

"Shirley! Isn't that Claude?"

I followed to where she was pointing to. She was right, that ram certainly was Claude, my heartbreaker. I was going to return now after grunting for a short while. Oh gosh, he was actually coming to me to see me. As he moved towards me, he carried all of the ewes' gazes lovingly looking at him.

"Bonjour, Shirley, how are you?"

I performed the mandatory double kiss on each cheek to get all the ewes who were looking open mouthed. Something I learnt and repeatedly did since five years ago with this gentle-ram.

"I'm very well, Claude, fancy seeing you here."

As no excitement was felt about seeing him, I kept my answers in a monotone capacity. Hopefully, Claude would gage that.

"Mon Cherie we must go to a bar for you to tell me all I've missed!"

This sentence made me question exactly what he wanted me to say. From the day you cancelled our wedding until now? No, thank you, unless you want to offer me glasses of wine.

"Well, that's a lovely offer but I'm busy tonight with friends so maybe another time."

I spun to make my way up the hill to my spot before I heard him yell, "TOMORROW?!"

He sounded desperate to me, but he delivered those words with a look that held a vat full of naughtiness. An honest look I fell in love with.

I wandered back to my spot with Charlene not that far behind me, so expected to my questions to her regarding her beau Barry.

"Shirley, do tell on what just happened with Claude, I hope he wasn't mean to you?"

Annoyingly, Claude was very nice and becoming to me. What a dick.

"Claude was all right, he asked me to join him some time in the future for a glass but I'm uncertain he will keep to that."

Charlene became too excited regarding this and I thought if only she knew what I went through. The false promises he made to me in hindsight made it obvious he would buckle out of our marriage.

"He's definitely more than all right, Shirl, he looked ravishing and sounds amazing, all of the ewes in the area properly swooned over him. You might enjoy the wine evening you're going to have."

'Shut up, Charlene!' Is what I wanted to say but didn't as I didn't want to break her heart as she probably believed in happily ever after and Claude was the one for me until eternity. Just like how she probably feels about Barry now. If she pipes up about Claude, I will savagely serve her the details of when relationships go wrong.

"I believe we have both moved on and the last I heard about him was that he was happily living in France. I haven't got a clue as to why he's rocked around here, and I don't really care."

Instant deflation occurred for Charlene, so I gave a half smile. She seriously cannot expect me to be happy after my ex-fiancé invited me to join him for a couple of jars. One more chance, not to say anything Charlene just remain quiet and your dream of a perfect wedding and happily-ever-after exists. One more chance.

"I just think, this Claude definitely deserves to have a meeting with you, I mean he has come all the way from France to see you, so you could at least offer your company."

My hooves were stamped. I definitely gave her the chance to remain muted, but she chose to speak. Well, this has confirmed for me to use the meanness of words up to the highest level. I took a deep breath and felt my wind pipe and voice box begin to rumble, I took a deep breath.

"Claude has been the worst C-word of all the other rams I've gone out with. He didn't appreciate going out with me after work or at weekends. In fact, he would just use the line, 'We'll just go out at the weekend' multiple times, something I have used in order to go out in public with him, but did he do that? No. I was once told he had another flame even though he had gone down on one knee previously. Eternal love? I don't think so."

Charlene nodded along with my anti-Claude speech. I hope it didn't cause too many chips of her dreams, but I was being honest. Claude would not stand by anything he says, he couldn't even go to a night he had arranged himself. Nothing, so trot off, Claude, there is nothing to see here.

The more I thought about how rubbish my ex was, the more I appreciated Richard. His look at me when he wanted to bow down and get his piece of paper signed by the famous Barry was just perfect strip of visuals I replayed repeatedly. Not like anything Claude has ever done for me. In fact, Claude leaving our home shutting the front door with a slam could be used as a reminder not to trust anyone.

This saddened me as I do believe Richard could make me believe in love and true marriage. I am still hopeful that my vegan dedication pays off for Richard to fall head over hooves in love with me.

Charlene arranged for when I should come to her barn to-night.

"I'll bring wine for us all to guzzle? Don't worry, the wine is clearly labelled vegan, something you two would probably worry about."

Chapter 10

Only when I had a moment to look around the interior from my seating position, I noticed the interior of the place I had been to many times. The massive mirror where we often adorned ourselves with makeup looked the same as before, but the potted plants and flowers were new additions. The place oozed thoughtfulness with calmness. I appreciated that, something I should try in my bedroom, although I severely doubted, I would actually change anything. That would mean putting work in.

The atmosphere between Charlene and Barry was wonderful. There wasn't any over the top kissing and it was relaxed and lovely to see the hoof touching between the pair of them. After eating the main rainbow salad which made me realise my journey to making dinner of sweet potato and beans a complete last place entrant in any cooking competition. Complete marvel at whoever was the chef on what I just ate. I'd put money on that it was Barry who oversaw what just went down my trachea and into my stomach bag with the upmost deliciousness.

Barry leaned over the table to ask, "How did you like the food, Shirley? Charlene told me you enjoy finding new vegan foods to eat." Should I make him aware of my excitement when I found out about pasta being vegan or just quietly nod and smile? I chose to silently nod and smile, to which Barry clapped his hooves and winked at me saying,

"That's great! I'll put this recipe on my website. Thanks, Darl!"

I gave an internal tut at him. Just a casual harmless sexism from him but a nice message, none the less. No wonder he had half of the restaurateurs lining up to get his autograph. Maybe I should ask him about what I should be cooking at home.

"You know it is really easy to create quick dinners, I'm sure Charlene has told you about some."

Barry said and looked at Charlene and smiled. I wish Richard was here as I felt really by myself and a true gooseberry. At least, I would have someone gorgeous to look at whilst in the dulls of conversation. With this thought, Barry suddenly asked me, "Why are you a vegan, Shirley?"

To that, I wanted to scream multiple swearwords and ask him if it would really make me happy to say goodbye to cakes, doughnuts and lots of fun. The main reasoning was to get the heartthrob of the farm to fall in love with me. I felt I couldn't give that sort of answer as I'm guessing he would have wanted more. I just fell into the trap of what every other gives.

"For my health really, Barry."

It hit me hard to fall into the stereotype, but I couldn't have given him a detailed reason behind what was behind going vegan.

Barry loudly said, "Oh that's interesting, Shirley because Charlene told me you wanted to go vegan because you wanted to go out with my mate, Richard?"

Wow, what a dick thing to say. I've gone back to where I've started from with him. Yeah, my new best friend going out with him has lessened my hatred of him but not by too much. Did Barry really have to heighten his tone of voice at the end of the question? Well, in fact questioner Barry, yes you have been fed credible information on the reason why I went vegan. I am not going to protest what he has said to me. I can however be grumpy at Charlene for spilling my own love gossip to her boyfriend.

"Yes, Barry, you are correct."

"I can mention something to Rich if you want? I think he's not available to date now as he has a girlfriend. Sorry."

Ouch, Barry, ouch! I needed to say something about what I witnessed at the noodle bar. I should say something, shouldn't I?

"Don't say anything about me to Richard yet, Barry! Please don't say anything about me at all! Yes?"

I felt the nervous and desperateness in my vocals when I spoke with Barry. Hopefully, he would have understood my need.

Barry just sighed at me and let out a couple of laughter bursts. I screwed up my face and raised one eyebrow implying I didn't know what he found funny.

"It's all right, Shirl, I won't mention anything about you to him. I promise you, I promise you that."

The earnest smile he gave me was a bit creepy to be honest, but I smiled back. Surely, it was time for me to reveal what I saw of Richard's girlfriend entering Ronald's? Yes, I believe that time was now.

"Richard's girlfriend just walked straight into Ronald's that night when we all went to the noodle bar. How can Richard not instantly dump her?"

Barry gave a small laugh and changed the shape of his lips to mimic but made a small cough to ready himself to speak.

"Well, Shirley, Richard doesn't need to only date vegans, that's not a rule! She can eat whatever she wants and be his girlfriend! I'm sorry to tell you that. You are on the right course to get his attention though, if you fancy a bit of weight loss, you're on the right diet because you're not eating any saturated fat. That's meat and dairy by the way."

It was Charlene's turn to *pfft*.

"You don't need to lose any weight sweetheart! You have a perfect figure, one that I'm jealous of."

I didn't agree with her there, but I did give myself a cuddle in my mind.

"Is it really true about the weight loss thing? I must be skinny by now because I've been vegan for almost three weeks!"

Barry grunted and sat upright to make a mini speech. Again.

"Veganism isn't a weight loss tool. It's a happy side effect of eating food that is perfect for our bodies. You told me that you're aware of the Gbombs? If you stick with that then you'll meet all of your nutritional needs and not eat nothingness to ward off hunger."

That was a good mini speech by Barry, I'll give him that. It became clear why he was such a vegan rock star. I was almost giving him a round of applause but held off and gave him a smile and nod. It was my turn to enter conversation, Barry held the conversational limelight for too long.

"Here's a question, Barry; what meal would you want to eat? I know you'll reel out lots of information on reasons why you shouldn't eat it, but humour me please?"

I bet he'll go for a T-bone steak because most rams feel eating steaks boost their manliness. Or maybe a sirloin even though that's a boring steak to go for in the steak options.

"Okay, here is something I would have if were duly pardoned from veganism, garlic shallots."

Bull shit, Barry! I doubt that entirely! Fish food? Really? Not even a steak or a sausage? I asked you to humour me but not make it a joke answer.

Charlene just sighed and rubbed his forearm with her hoof. I needed to get some sense of clarity after the 'garlic shallots' answer. It was time to call my new best friend out. This was the least I could do after she was caught out sharing something, I thought was private with her boyfriend. Who inappropriately used it against me somehow?

"Charlene, didn't we both bitch about us being vegans and didn't want to be like the 'namby-pamby' vegans who meditated and prayed a lot? You even told me the joke about finding out who the vegan is at a party is that you say nothing because the vegan finds you. Remember that, do you, Charlene? You weren't so innocent a vegan as you make out."

After saying that I sat down. Standing up always gives me a sense of power. Unfortunately, Charlene took my shouting to heart and selfishly started to cry. My bedroom was calling out to me, so I thanked my friends and retired gracefully. My retirement didn't miss the odour of baked vegan friendly chocolate cake which almost made me reverse back to the table. I didn't, of course, because by doing so would ruin my graceful retirement style I was hoping to achieve. Only a few more trots and I would be in my bedroom.

"Bonsoir, Shirley?"

No, it couldn't have been, but it certainly was. Did Claude really think I'd enjoy my ex who I made perfectly clear I wanted to keep him as an ex.

"Yeah, fuck off, Claude."

I pushed my arm away to make a backwards wave, an action I hoped would class as a solemn goodbye but oh no, Claude was walking to the side of me. A tactic he always used to do back when we were going out. A tactic that I didn't care for and found it annoying in all honesty.

With his arm forcibly linked to my arm, I felt the need to squawk.

"What the fuck are you doing? We both know we don't want this so why are you holding my arm?"

My eyes met his and the part of my brain reserved for loving Claude feelings experienced a flash.

Objection of good feelings for Claude sparked into action. The front door being slammed shut as he left to go to another place. The wedding we were happy to plan, the moments I was left by myself thinking he would join me. All those half hours I staunchly waited in whatever weather to see my Claude come into my vision to make it all right. They were objectionable memories all right. Now, I just needed to signal for him to leave.

"Is there any reason you're hanging around me, do you actually want to be deployed?"

We've spoken about this before, in a joke. This joke made us feel the same creatures as when he lived with me. My boiling contempt started to cool.

Chapter 11

The night that passed was remarkably enjoyable as we shared stories of when we once had fun. It was only when we had both finished talking that Claude brought his head closer to mine and said, "one last time?" I gallantly pushed him away from me and sneered, "No, thank you." I thought about the times when I screamed and mentioned deportation, but he always laughed at me and straggled my wool giving me a peck on my forehead.

When I finally touched down on my mattress with my duck down duvet, I slept perfectly. Charlene has certainly got a good ram, if he could effortlessly construct a meal I had last night, then I'd marry him myself. Once his wool is sorted out. It's too eighties rock band for my liking.

Despite promising myself to skip to the farm for work, I felt that languorously walking to the entrance of the farm seemed fitting. Must try skipping tomorrow.

When I fully stood at my position, I had a sense of my gaydar flickering for no fathomable reason. My phone was innocently tucked away in my bag, I thought it best to retrieve it and send a message to William to see if he and Steve would want a drink at the pub for a chinwag.

I allowed myself two minutes of working and then thought it best to send a message to William before break time. I needed to know how best to plan my rest timetable.

'We are not feeling going to the pub but want to go to the tea-rooms down the road if you fancy coming with us?'

I've seen the tea rooms down the road from the Red Lion before but have never passed the front door so this will be an exciting meeting with both William and Steve within all of the regency decorated walls. I didn't have clue as to who king George was about, but the restaurant owners loved him and plastered him everywhere. I'll wiki him when I have the time. I'll just put in 'King George' and that will bring him up.

It felt marvellous drinking tea out of quaintly decorated tea cups and I felt like Alice in wonderland, sipping green tea whilst sticking my little finger up. Steve smiled at me and said, "How do you feel, madam? This is a much nicer drinking spot than the pub we think." Whilst he spoke, he circled his trotters lightly on William's thigh. My jealousy spectrum was lit at a three level which meant I didn't feel the need to grunt as it was wonderful to see them both happy, I only wished for myself to have a partner too.

When I mentioned this fact to the couple, they instantly roared with pleasure. Steve clapped his hooves. This was the first time I noticed his campiness when he said, "Oh yes darling, we need to set you up with a single ram we know."

This made me giggle internally. Who on earth could be single on the farm? I thought that Charlene would have made me aware of any singletons but sat here with William and Steve made me realise that I were to go closer to the singleton stream. This would be exciting, should I make requests as to what this mysterious ram looks like? It wouldn't cause offence and will make my cupids happy. Right, I should begin with my specification.

"He has to have mousy wool colour. Good looking in the modern-day value. Umm, maybe have good teeth with a strong jaw line?"

The guys laughed, and William broke off to say, "You're quite specific in your demands aren't you, Shirley?"

I gave a small tittering. I didn't mention the vegan thing as I remembered what Barry said. Being vegan doesn't mean you have to stick with a vegan. It would be cool if he was though.

"So how long have you been single for if you don't mind me asking?"

Steve's question was unexpected but completely understandable. Claude dumped me five years ago and I haven't had much action since. Yes, I've had brief kisses, but nothing was incredible to me. Nothing as good as Claude, his kissing was quite amazing.

Why was I walking towards Claude's barn? I really didn't like him.

Claude reached me in the walking line to his barn. For an unknown reason, I made sure I didn't make any eye contact with him as I knew I'd fall into the dip again with him, of actually fancying him again. Something I will not do.

William rushed over to me and had clearly run a great distance as he was out of breath and took a quick breath to say, "Okay, Shirley, we've had a discussion as to who we're going to set you up with, have you ever heard of a ram called Justin?"

I racked my brain to think if I've ever met a Justin, this was something that I didn't believe I did. I'll be happy to meet this Justin. I needed to know more of this mysterious ram. The longer I didn't know about him, the more I became interested in him.

"When can I meet this Justin? I hope he's near-by, I've got a scary suspicion he's waiting behind the corner or something."

William laughed and gave me an honest shake of head.

"Oh, that's a shame. I wonder where this creature called Justin is at this very moment. You guys probably know this, do you?"

William shook his head and genuinely smiled at me.

"Justin is an ex-policeman who is wanting to get some extra work to tide him over for Christmas. He fills your quota that you set out earlier and could make you happy."

This synopsis of Justin was quite pleasing, I wonder where we are going to meet.

It was as if Steve read my mind and swooped in with a comment,

"How do you fancy meeting at the water sculpture down the road. That is where William and I first kissed, so I hope it will shed some wonder dust on you both."

The cheesy grin with eyebrow raising was nice because it didn't over fill my metre of twee-ness.

I smiled back and turned to head to my barn where I could think about this Justin. It would be good if I had Charlene's opinion on this, but she had disappeared for some time away from me. In all, it was over two days and I wanted to talk rubbish with her. She was after all my new best friend. Surely, she should have instant dismissal for not being around me being set up with this 'Justin'.

As I reached into my bag, I could feel an overwhelming French presence, looking over my shoulder and waited for him to say something, because he had always done so in the past. Probably something dramatic and asking a question. That he'll want me to answer immediately.

"Ma bon, Cherie Shirley, how are you?"

Even though I lived with his accent for years I still get a front bottom fuzz over it. I will reply but boringly and unattractively. Maybe I'll sniff and muck around with my nostrils to make me appear unattractive. This was something I thought Claude felt when he dumped me.

"Yeh, I'm good, cheers, Claude."

He shuffled where he was standing. Something didn't seem right with him. I kept shouting at myself to not care but he looked in a bad way.

"I just wanted to ask you something that you could help me with. I know you hate me, but I just wanted to talk to you inside."

This was an odd thing to say from him, normally he keeps everything locked up inside and doesn't ask for anything. This prompted my overarching caring for the guy. I gave him an innocent pat on the back.

Claude over expressed his appreciation with a prolonged grunt. Memories came flooding back to me whilst he made that sound, it tended to lead into romantic time. Never again. The more times I said this, the more I'll believe it.

"So yes, my question…" to which I

He leaned towards me and cuddled my hooves instantly moved away from.

The talking was muted but he looked up at me with sorrowful eyes, the same eyes he had when he proposed to me. Deep brown and beautiful. I should really turn away and study something else that was in my room. Oh, the starling sculpture that was placed on my shelf, I can really study that.

"You are the only ewe on this planet who I could spend the rest of my life with, you must have felt the same. I'm sorry for leaving you but over the past few years I've been wanting to turn back time and really appreciate you for being you. Oh, sweet angel, I was an overwhelming idiot for not appreciating every drop of you."

Claude almost made me feel something for him then, but only a scratch worth. Nothing to get worried about.

"Well, that is lovely to hear, Claude, but you are five years too late. My heart has been well and truly broken and there is no entrance for you to enter again. Never."

I had to give myself an internal fist bump because that was a mean roasting. Something that I enjoyed doing.

His growl was not needed so I tutted at him, what a waste of oxygen to growl like that.

"Do you want money, Claude? Is that why you're hanging around my barn?"

Claude shirked away from me when I said that, now is the time when he gets annoyed about something and blows his top.

"NO, Shirley, I just want you to know how deeply sorry I am for hurting you. If possible and I don't want to apply pressure or force you in anyway but can I sleep in your bed with you?"

Chapter 12

I did not sleep in my usual bed last night. The groan of my misdemeanour was powerful. How could I do something so stupid with my dastardly ex? The smoothness of calm was welcomed by me when I acknowledged the fact that Justin had no idea that I partook in sexual intercourse with my ex-boyfriend. This could serve as an act of nightly practice in my favour if anything romantic were to occur between Justin and me.

Claude was straight out of my door as soon as daylight occurred. The feeling of being hurt was soon to be quashed when I remembered when he did the same whilst we were going out. Him, leaving me this morning, seemed a minor rudeness I could roll over and pull up my duvet. Bye-bye you, pathetic ram, you were good practice, but I hope to never see you again. Bye-bye.

When I was completely alone in my solitude, I came across a thought of how I got into meeting Claude in the first place.

I was sitting in the pub with my old friend, Mike, who I scarcely contact anymore. The last I heard of his travels was him moving to south London. That was it, although the memories still lived on. I doubt I will ever be in contact with Mike again, not now, that I'm miles away on the southern coast. That's over one hundred and fifty miles away. Or something like that.

It was two-thousand and six when I focussed what I wanted from life. First of the things I wanted was a dating life, because that would probably bring a boyfriend and then marriage. It was all settled in my mind. I just needed help to start the first steps into the dating world. If only I could blurt into the group chat about getting dumped by my fiancé who I met from these discussions being had.

My Flashback:

"Yes, Shirley! Good for you! What's your Ideal ram? What are you looking for?"

I sat back and thought. Despite placing effort on the announcement of my dating ambitions, I failed to contemplate the fundamental aspects of my dating.

"Well, he'd have to be muscly. Be a teacher, fireman or policeman. With blue eyes, he'd have to have blue eyes. He'd have to play sport, like rugby or cricket. But I'd take football. And most of all, he'd have blonde wool."

Mike looked at me puzzlingly. I sipped my drink and raised my eyebrows imploring him to speak.

"Shirley you've just described a carbon copy of Chris. Nearly everything you've said as your ideal ram, matches Chris. Except you didn't mention doctor as an ideal profession because he is one. I think you need to widen your horizons. If you want a good place to start, I'd suggest online dating."

Jade nodded, "Yes! Mike's right. I can set up your profile! Can you remember how many dates I used to get offered when I did it?"

"Yes, but you never actually went on any dates. You just enjoyed looking at their pictures and emailing them."

Jade blushed and I felt a sharp shock of guilt and instantly regretted highlighting her low confidence in the dating world.

I quickly felt the impulse to belittle myself as an act of atonement.

"Sorry, Jade but I'm not too sure about it. I don't think I have the confidence to actually go and meet someone I met online."

Jade smiled and offered her help with creating a dating profile. I enquired whether it was necessary to give my age.

"I don't think my 28 years should be displayed; I might as well emblazon my profile with the words 'Mutton Alert'."

As per usual, Mike pointed out the sensibilities of display-
ing an age and offered encouragement that 28 is young and
the best years are still ahead of me. I could enjoy feeling re-
laxed with Mike's perception of age due to his ten years sen-
iority over both me and Jade, due to his being part of the flock
our current farmer inherited.

"All right, I'll give my age. Jade, I'd be very grateful for
your help but let's not rush into anything too soon, I'm quite
shy to meet a stranger from online."

Jade smiled, and I felt at ease; I'd adequately returned to
the equilibrium whilst maintaining an air of timidity. That was
until Mike scoffed,

"Rubbish, Shirley! You have more than enough confi-
dence for online dating. Give it a go. That's how I met my new
flame."

I really hoped Mike has had success in whatever he
wanted to do. He might have married that 'flame' that he
spoke about those years ago. He was a ram who would have
been against me having affairs with Claude. I could just imagine his head shaking at me as though he was some sort of
life manager. He was someone who always thought he was
better than the farmer.

The more times I thought about Claude, the more down I
became. I've not come needing to find a positive thought to
balance my equilibrium. The happiest thoughts I could have
at this moment was about this Justin. I altered this rule to
mean; I could think about Claude if is bad regarding him. For
example, if any evidence comes to my attention about where
he went after leaving my barn. In fact, I don't want to know
where he went, just knowledge, I am soon to be set up with
Justin.

The uplifting thoughts regarding what outfit I should wear
on this date overtook any other thoughts. The make-up needed
to match my outfit. Charlene would be the best to talk me
through that, but she is currently AWOL at the moment. I really should direct my thoughts as to how to win her back as a
new best friend. I will say sorry for just leaving the dinner

party she'd set up after a pointless cross of lines. Thinking of which, she still has bottle of wine that I took to the dinner. She should be apologetic to me! I will ignore that and will not mention this wine stealing tabasco. In fact, we could have a wine evening where we could design my aesthetic look for the Justin date. As nothing much was happening in town, I decided to walk home. As my barn was next door to Charlene's barn, I decided to pop by and aid the tension we were experiencing. Supreme societal negotiations you might call it, but adequate pre-date care is what I would call it.

She spent over the amount of time was needed from the first rung of the doorbell but I was ready with a grin.

"Oh, hello, Shirley! What are you doing around here? Anything I can help you with?"

That was a cringe-worthy hello. Did I appreciate her language? Not really but I could with her help with the incredibly good make-up like she did when we met William at the pub. How best to tactually put this to her? Maybe overwhelm her with praise so she will abide by any question you give her. I think that's the best way of talking.

"Actually, Charlene, there is a favour to ask you. You know how you did my make up the other night when we met William at the Red Lion? Well, I honestly thought you did my make up to a professional standard and I just wondered if you could do the same again on me. I have a date soon and want to look gorgeous. So, could you help?"

Charlene smiled and made a way for me to enter the barn. I took that action as a yes. When I passed the kitchen, I could see Barry flipping grilled vegetables in a sauce pan. I was directed to sit on the hessian sofa.

"Tell me who you spent last night with, Shirley. When I checked the street before locking up, I think I saw you, arm in arm with Claude. Were my eyes correct? Did Claude stay over? I thought you hated him."

I really wanted to keep her voice speaking to me as I was obviously rubbish being by myself.

"Well, it was wonderful talking about past experiences that made us laugh. We did have a kiss."

She wasn't buying it.

"What happened after that? I doubt you left it as only that, did you have nookie? Just be honest with me, Shirley."

Now this was a tricky answer to deal with, it posed a big angry argument if I get it wrong. If I said, we did nothing and just laid in bed was a lie and could be sussed easily and ruin my planned make-up assistant working with me. However, if I told the brutal truth about what happened and he passed me in various shapes, I didn't realise I could do and was more flexible than what I thought I was. I could always mention he left me when it was daylight to build sympathy and ensure she would do my make-up.

"So, how did you leave things with Claude? Are you wanting to get back together with him?"

A sigh escaped my mouth and I thought about what I was going to say that neatly wraps it all up. This needed to be a wise paragraph that's not too short or too long.

"Things were left amicable on both sides as we both real-ised life was better by ourselves when we didn't have the wed-ding rings on our fingers."

I gave a smile, but Charlene squished her face up. It was time to bring in the big drama to make her know I didn't want anything to do with him anymore at all.

"When I woke up, it was daylight and he had disap-peared."

That line should do it, hopefully she'd agree to be my make-up artist. An added short sentence would be enough to clench it.

"I just want to find someone who will love me."

There, that line will work.

Chapter 13

After attaining Charlene's acceptance of being my fashion designer for my date with Justin, I felt confident of the dress I bought at the charity shop. Unfortunately, I don't think I won the charity clothing lottery as there are no labels on the dress at all. The dress does look exceptionally good on me, so I salute the vegan gods. All I need now is for the date to be brought forward so I can show it off without causing any food staining to happen because I doubted highly to keep the dress pristine. I've already saved countless animal lives adopting the V diet, so didn't want to be too fussed about not spilling drinks or food mouthfuls on it.

Whilst I was preparing to leave for work, my eyes danced around the ring, the shop robot told me to buy. The sales assistant also told me it really suited my eye colour and dress colour, I had just purchased. With those selling credentials, I needed to purchase the ring. I wonder if Justin would appreciate it. I can imagine he would, as he strikes me as a classy sheep, one who probably has a downstairs wine cellar, plays golf at the weekends and loves opera. I really hope Justin isn't like that. How could I possibly chat on a level playing field? He could be a vegan, I could chat about that with him. My phone buzzed to attention and saved me from designing what Justin is like, I've had bad experiences, believing blind dates could have been models. All of them weren't. Justin could however be a model, he's being set up by two very good-looking rams, one being William, a part time model who is gorgeous, so obviously Justin will be of a similar ilk.

"Hey, Shirley, how are you?"

I knew that voice, it sounded mightily familiar that a quick flip to look backwards wouldn't hurt.

"Steve! What you doing here? Aren't you working on the adjacent farm?"

Well, that was a shock to see, it was only a couple of days since we met up in the tea shop where the idea for a date for myself was floated.

"Yes, I am gorgeous, just thought I'd better check with you if you are still on for a date with Justin on Saturday?"

An answer was needed but I didn't want to rush anything out and needed to sound cool. Should I tell Steve, Justin has been on my mind nonstop and that I've bought a dress that makes me look utterly gorgeous? Not to forget the classical ring that cost five times more money? Granted the dress was of charity shop prices. Just be cool, Shirley, don't sound too excited.

"Yes, Saturday is good with me."

Effortless answering. I was proud of me then. I wondered what Steve would say as an acknowledgement. Something which I hoped he would do. For some reason, I had a rush imagining he would say nothing and just trot off. He didn't seem like the guy to do that, he could actually be a decent ram, doing his best for his friend called Justin. Would it be strange to ask him about Justin's credentials?

"Well, that is excellent, Justin is really looking forward to your date."

Asking about those credentials suddenly felt the best way to continue this conversation. "I am also really looking forward to our date."

No, I wanted to know more about this ram who I'm seeing on Saturday. I want to know more about his facial measurements, his hair colour and his smile. What questions should I ask to attain this information? Steve stepped in to answer all of these questions.

"Is it all right if we have a selfie together? Justin wants a picture of you, but I can't find any photo of you sober, in most of them you look drunk pulling gruesome faces, but I know you're better than that, so can I take selfie now? Don't worry you look gorgeous au naturel!"

My photos online are terrible. I blame Claude for those as we just lived on wine in those days. I never spent glamorising time on myself so no wonder I looked pathetic on a night out.

Of course, I will have a selfie with him, if I didn't then I'd be painting myself off as an ultimate diva who only takes shots in the evenings when it's dim. That actually was a good photographic time but I daren't say anything to prolong the waiting of snaps. He'd get frustrated but this might mean that Justin would be too. Oh, I better just get this over with.

"Okay, let's take a selfie, but can you give me a photo of Justin too?"

Steve grinned, this was either going to be a cause of procrastination or a handover of images of Justin himself. Both options were bearable, so I grinned back.

"Okay, if you come and stand next to me, I'll take a selfie of us both?"

The direct method of self-photography was an incredible feat. The movement of which had obviously been practiced before. When the shots were looked over, it wreaked of professionalism. He must have put on one of those 'effects' because the entire shot looked too good. It looked as though it was out of a glossy fashion magazine. I told him but he just shrugged and said, I go out with a fashion model so am aware of how to take the best shots.

I checked on the phone holding the selfie. It hadn't changed its position on my palm. What a wonderful photographic session I've had. I'd pay good money to own that. The more I studied it, the more I wanted to be next to Justin. My trust in William and Steve was blindingly unshakeable. He'd better be the ram of my dreams. I thought it best to push for Justin's image.

"Umm, well, I have some images of him but they're old now, like five or six years old. He looks exactly the ones taken on my phone."

I sensed there was something interesting he was going to say on the matter. I mean, how could he change the way he looks after five, six years? Unless he's put on weight, maybe that's right and he has ballooned himself to such a degree that he has become unrecognisable. I was prepared for Steve to deliver me this news and nod apologetically with thoughts of *Poor guy, he must have fallen into the cheese trap* spinning around my mind. I could easily empathise with him as after I went through my third break up with Claude, I discovered the pull of crisps and ice cream to nurse me being alone.

"Well, he does look the same but annoyingly he has weight. Not so much that he's skeletal but he has lost weight."

This is interesting. What a peculiar thing to say. Did he believe I was an ordering witch as to be disappointed with Justin being a few pounds overweight? From what I've seen William and Steve have achieved a great cupid service. The rest is down to me, making myself a glamorous princess to meet her prince charming. There was only a matter of hours before I am stood on the allocated meeting spot. That reminded me that I wasn't totally ready for my dating catwalk as I haven't discussed the hair style that I should have with Charlene. My thoughts are for a rough curling with volume and holding spray all around my head. Yes, I will say exactly this when I next see my new best friend as I believed this was something she should be notified of.

Two kisses on each cheek were shared with Steve as he left my farm. It didn't take me long before I noticed a white sheep in the distance bounding left to right. When I halted my grazing work, I realised that it was Charlene who was making a fuss about walking in a straight line. She sped up her pace when we made eye contact. I held pity for her as I know she wasn't the fittest of ewes.

"Shirley! Richard's girlfriend has run away! It's all a bit confusing at Burley. Some are saying she's run away with someone else! Nobody knows who this someone could be, but I will let you know as soon as I know."

This was exciting news, coming from the bounding white cloud who calls herself my new best friend. So, this is an interesting romantic spot to be in. I am definitely going to see this Justin but have Richard in the background. I was looking forward to learn about Chloe's decision to up sticks and leave the best ram on the farm. I'll look forward to hearing about the romantic gossip hot off the press by Charlene.

Charlene's face lit up and it looked as though she wanted to explode. Her right hoof flapping certainly gained my attention. What was she doing? I hoped she would put me out of my misery and tell me what was on her tongue. For the past three years I've known her, she had always enjoyed knowing things I'm unaware of.

"I know how her lover could be! It's just clicked with me, you know the ram who you had a nightly escapade?"

I knew exactly who she was talking about, but I didn't want to think about what she was thinking. Claude and I had a wonderful time together and to think he was the callous of the callous, I already knew him of was sickening.

"I believe your Claude left your barn in the morning to search out where Chloe was. Thinking about it, it makes sense they were drawn to each other. They are French so could probably speak in the sexy sounding language. Yes, that's it, everything is clicking in for me now!"

The slow nod goodnight I gave Charlene was saddened by the realisation of it actually being a fact.

Chapter 14

The morning began with the remembrance of what I learnt about my ex-fiancé's positioning around this farm. When I had removed the oats, I left soaking in almond milk overnight, I grabbed the nuts that were available to me and then had a chef moment when I chucked over the uneaten seeds we had with our Thai takeaway. I should be recognised as a masterful chef as I have quite often used my cheffing vegan knowledge to create mouth-watering dishes. Barry told us that most vegan food tastes great because that's the type of food we should eat. I told him not everybody wants to be told to eat something they don't like. I for myself, did not like mushrooms because I thought they looked ugly but now I love them. Probably because of the vegan gods casting a spell on me to like them. The sprinkling of seeds on top of my porridge, made me look a professional chef.

My phone buzzed with a message. It was my day off which I had dedicated towards preparing myself for the date with Justin. Who could possibly be waiting to contact me? I would place money on a bet it is Charlene.

'*Hi Sweetheart! How are you feeling about tonight's date?*'

Kerching! I'm the winner, it is my new best friend contacting me. Just politely adding a bit of pressure to the date.

'*Hey yes, Char, I'm very excited! Are you all right to do my hair as well as make up?*'

She would have definitely said yes with excitement. I'll give her a second to reply.

'*Oh my god, yes!*'

That was to be expected but it did give me a friendly and excited buzz in my belly. This will actually happen. I am going to woo Justin and we will live happily ever after. Unless, he proposes and leaves me living without a fiancé like what Claude achieved. I scolded myself for even thinking about the nasty ram. I will think no more regarding him.

Within ten minutes, since opening my barn door, Charlene unloaded her big sack full of instruments and make up bags. My newly purchased bottle of red was calling to me to be collected, so I darted away from where Charlene had placed me.

As I left, I whispered, "Wine," and gave a wink. I did not appreciate her giving me side headed treatment. When I sneaked in to the kitchen, I thought it best to creep back to the make-up boudoir with the bottle and glasses.

"Okay, Shirley, let's do your hair style first and then we'll work on your make-up yeah?"

I nodded hastily and tugged away from the plastic wrapping surrounding the wine with my teeth. When the bottle lid was naked of plastics, it was free to be poured into the wineglasses I had prepared sitting on the table. When I poured out two glasses, I looked up at my make-up artist, who was scarily studying my face. It made me become worried as if I had done something wrong or maybe she had seen my freckles and were matching them up to make a shape or something. My freckles are too weak to easily cast a glance at my face to achieve this shape construction.

Charlene drew a breath to start speaking. This would be good to hear, despite not blocking my ear canals, I thought it best to have a sip of my wine and place it on the table.

"Did you know that your right eye was slightly higher than your left?"

Well, that was news to me and guaranteed she wouldn't get a tip.

"Well, thank you for that insight, Charlene. I hope your eye observation won't hinder you whilst doing my make-up. Maybe I should push my right eye to match the level of my left eye?"

Hopefully, she will chuckle at that statement as I was of course, mocking myself.

"Oh, that would be cool if you can."

There wasn't even a hint of a chuckle. An internal eyeroll promptly happened after she uttered it. She was my new best friend, but I shouldn't be in charge of educating her.

"Okay, can you pass me that brush over there and I'll brush out all of the knots of your hair."

That was a double insult giving as I've learnt about my left eye being slightly higher than my right and my wool was horrendously matted. I considered about what the trio of insults could be.

"You can still see where you dyed your hair green that time when you went to a Halloween party five years ago. It's amazing that it's still there. How many baths do you have?"

There, that would be the trio.

Feeling the yanking of the hairbrush, struggling to run down my wool effortlessly like a distant dream, every time a new ball of knots were found a signal of rudeness. She didn't even offer an apology when she caused my head to fly backwards and I let out a yelp. Rude.

"So, what are you looking for when you meet Justin?"

A true love would be an embarrassing thing to say but that was the truth. If I played it down then anything would seem like a bonus.

"Just someone nice to talk to."

That was epically taking it down. Charlene had nothing more to say and would presumably work on my hairstyle, without causing anymore hair brushing yelping.

"Nah, Shirl, you want someone who has a bit of flavour to them. Claude had lots of spice when you met him. So, you said."

From those words, I realised I needed to teach Charlene not only English but a large dose of how to be tactful. Saying things like that about my ex was not necessary, especially when I was hoping to come across spice when meeting Justin.

"Yes, Claude was indeed flavourful, but do I really want to meet another Claude? Really?"

Charlene physically shirked her body when I said that.

I genuinely felt sorry for her to do that. Hearing the words leave my mouth, I felt strengthened. I wasn't wrong in my belief, I didn't want a carbon copy of Claude. I felt like patting myself on the back when I thought that. It must have been over twenty minutes since Charlene started attacking my hair, so I thought it best to enquire about my hairstyling.

"Are you all right, Charlene? There's been over a minute since you've brushed my wool and I've become accustomed to yelping every ten seconds, I feel something has prevented you from carrying on. Here, have this glass of wine. I'll drink mine too and we'll spend a couple of minutes to have a break and recover. Me for the wool being plucked out of its routes and you to ease your wrist for repeated brushing against the matting."

Charlene smiled and raised her glass. I reciprocated and prepared myself for more pain. It was welcomed when Charlene started speaking as it prolonged the length of time until the brushing began.

"You know how I'm doing your make-up right? Shouldn't I be using those animal friendly products? Every ewe in the farm at Burley has those."

I really didn't want to snap at her or make herself feel down but I really thought it was important to say something.

"Yes, I really do think I should have animal friendly make-up, I don't want any animals to be harmed whilst testing is done on my makeup, neither do you, I assume, but I want to be made up using the make-up that's in my make-up bag. Has the make-up been tested on animals? I don't know but I know to find products that are not tested on animals in the future."

The meaningful words just kept coming out, so I rewarded myself with another pat on the back.

When she had placed the brush on the table and sat down, we both succinctly sighed. I brought my wineglass up to hers and said, "Cheers!"

The next date preparation was to be made up, I knew she was an expert in doing that for me so I could relax.

Chapter 15

I inputted the exact location of my date's meet into my phone and planned how I would get there elegantly emitting a sense of class and composure. When the map told me, I was half an hour away, I let out a shriek and started jogging, thinking the map was mistaken as it was only a small village and probably miscounted the distance. Whether it did give me the wrong time duration to the set meeting location, it was better to be early. Being early made me look cool and calm, just how I wanted Justin to think of me.

I kept looking down at my phone to check the map. 40 minutes until I reach the meeting location. How did that increase its timing? The massive internal eyeroll was called for after acknowledging the map timing was having a bit of a fluffy day as when I looked at it for the last time at it told me 52 minutes to destination. I started to jog just in case.

Standing at the desired meeting spot, I could hear someone puffing with quick footsteps to accommodate. My eyes focussed on where the sounds were being made from and to my pleasure it was Justin. So, I smiled and dipped my head to give a sense of outright elegance, something I yearned for at the beginning of my journey to here. It will be interesting to hear him speak because marrying up the image of him with the sound of his vocals could make me instantly fall in love with him.

"Hey! Shirley?"

He needed to take a few more breathes before beginning to talk again. Oh, and a ball of spit projected to the ground. This was not going to be the happy ever after date I thought it would be.

"I thought I wanted to be here early to meet you, but my map kept giving me lengthened time of travel duration each time I checked it. I thought it was probably best to run here."

I stewed over his speaking, he seemed quite warm hearted which was nice to hear. Should I mention that I too had a wacky duration time experience? I felt it best to offer sympathy and be internally smug I had reached here first. Yes, that seemed a better option to have.

"Did it take you long to get here? Where do you live?"

That was a worthy question because he could have come from somewhere miles away and not in this village. If he came from somewhere miles away, then it was stupid question and I will skim over the answer.

"I live relatively close to here, it's in Burley farm?"

No skimming over the answer was needed. I knew exactly where Burley Farm was as it was the farm adjacent to my own. My metre for happy ever after just shot up.

"Yes, I know Burley Farm, I'm amazed I haven't seen you around before."

Justin was quick to speak after I said that.

"I've seen you before! You might not have noticed me, but I definitely saw you."

Well, that had an element of sneakiness to it. Full body shake was needed after hearing that. That was a stalker-esque thing to say. I'll ignore those feelings and smiled.

"Where do you want to go? Do you want to go for a drink or meal?"

Superiority was made by me for saying that. Classy organised date was made out by me to add to Justin's impression. It would be interesting to hear his answer, hopefully, without the spitting.

"Umm, I reckon we should go for a meal. I've had a fast run so could really do with loading up on the lost calories."

I raised my eyebrows and nodded my head as if I was wholeheartedly agreeing. This was something I disagreed with as I wanted him to say 'drink'. Using my quick-thinking skills, I thought the restaurant's menu would offer alcohol so I would be satisfied with that.

"Do you know which restaurant you want to go to? The noodle bar on the high street is an excellent place to go in order to have a quick calorie-filled session?"

There, I made myself seem incredibly knowledgeable of the village high street. Hopefully, that would have satisfied what Justin was hoping for.

Justin gave a big wide grin and exemplified his feelings by giving me two thumbs up. I shot back a smile and beckoned him to walk with me along the street. He quickly trotted to be by my side which was a welcome feeling as most of the high street walking was done by me and Charlene, so it was nice to have a sense of masculinity next to me.

"Is it the place along here on the left?"

I bit my lip as the neon light clearly reads 'NOODLE BAR'. I nodded and smiled, it was too soon to make any assumptions about Justin's intelligence level. He might impress me when sat down.

My memory served me well as I could easily recall what I ordered the time before. When the waitress arrived at our table, I could effortlessly say my order. I checked to see if the wine I had ordered was vegan. That should be enough for us to chat about if we stumbled to come up with any topics of conversation. I really hoped he was a vegan because that would have made my eating life easier. Just having Charlene on the same eating page became a bit annoying and although it was great chatting to her vegan star boyfriend was nice and all I wanted was a new someone to chat do. I prepared myself with the typical vegan answers. If he dared even mention the word 'Protein', I'll give up on the happily ever premise.

"So, are you a vegan?"

Justin shot me quite a cutting look as if he wanted to make me feel pathetic. Those looks bolster me and I sat up straight.

"Yes, I am a vegan and am proud to be one. Give me the protein question."

He was obviously keen to hear my answer as he was looking at me as if he was a puppy waiting for orders. I had given him the next question to ask me so relaxed into my chair.

"Okay, I've always wanted to know this, where do you get your protein from?"

When he had finished talking, I saw a small flock gather to be seated at the back of the restaurant. It took me a couple of seconds to notice that Richard was amongst the crowd. It was nice seeing him alone without a girlfriend because despite me thinking there was no chance, we could ever meet romantically after vomit gate it was still nice to look at him.

"Do you know? Or is it a vegan secret thing?"

Oh, Justin was sat opposite me so I should answer.

"No, it's not a secret thing at all. Protein is made when the sun hits green food sources. So, the cows and other animals eat green food that have tons of protein. No wonder there's a thinking that meat is full of protein."

I glanced across to the table at the back. Just to check if Richard was still in that vicinity. He was.

"So, what's with the canine teeth? Surely they're there for us to eat meat?"

I wanted to answer him, but I was most interested in what was going on at the back of the restaurant. There was a lot of chatter about something. I'd best answer Justin quickly so I could investigate more with my eyes what was going on.

"Lots of herbivorous animals have canine teeth. The hippo and gorilla have huge ones, they help break down green protein sources. Not animals to prey on. They are not carnivores. The lions deserve canines, not us."

That would have adequately answered him. I could have told him about vegans having a higher level of protein in their blood than omnivores, but I didn't want to be smugger about that.

The noisy table at the back started to sing 'Happy Birthday' so that realised my wondering about what was going on. Before I could hear the name of the birthday song, the waitress blocked my view of staring at them.

"All of the alcohol that we have on the menu is vegan so the wine you've ordered is completely animal friendly."

The twee smile given didn't have to be done in such a way, but I smiled back. It was then when I thought about Justin. I wondered if he was okay.

"Are you all right, Justin? Eaten your fill of calories? The noodle dish that you have in front of you looks delicious!"

I gave my question with a sense of bounce. That would make him feel joyful as I should have been happier during this eating experience, but I was torn between the far table with the beautiful Richard on it and the table I was on. Justin was a good-looking ram but didn't possess that special something about his face like how Richard did. Maybe it was the fact I didn't splurge sick right in front of him. That must have been the magic love potion to make me fall in love even more due to the fact I gallantly kept churning out the sickness.

"Do you want me to get the bill?"

Awe, this was nice of Justin to say but I felt a big dollop of guilt spread over me. I hadn't wowed him the way I've done before other times on dates. During my date-athon after Claude dumped me, I went on lots of dates where I gladly accepted their gesture of paying for the bill, but not this time. I didn't belly laugh once and that was my signal to accept the payment gesture.

Justin got out of his chair and stood up. He started to walk and I assumed he had lost his way to the exit as he walked towards me. He bent down to look at me in the eye, I smiled at him because I thought he was joking about something but that was enough for him to kiss me.

Possibly the best kiss I've had in my life.

Chapter 16

My bed welcomed me back from my date with Justin and gave me the perfect place to relax and think about the expedition. It wasn't magnificent, but it was satisfactory. Yes, it didn't end up in a mad panic to get undressed and snog our faces off, but we left each other very well with a beautiful kiss. That seemed an unusual experience for me to have. My thinking was interrupted by my front barn door being opened. My new best friend was obviously wanting to have a briefing of my date with Justin.

"Soooo, how was it? Was he good looking?"

I was very appreciative of her words but didn't know how to answer her. Should I say he's good looking in a way but not as good looking as Richard? Do I even mention he was in the noodle bar at the same time? I might as well, she probably knows why there was quite a happy flock at the back of the restaurant.

"Well, it was nice, we went to the noodle bar for a meal. We had a kiss before we separated to go back to the farm."

Her mouth instantly shot open when I said that.

"Why are you surprised? Have I done something wrong?"

Charlene's sigh didn't fill me with happiness. I felt as though I did something wrong.

"No, nothing sweetheart! I just thought he might have stayed over, that's all."

My date experience obviously offended her in some way. She knows how I felt about sharing a bed with someone. Three dates were a minimum before the bedroom exercises. Sometimes, I altered this self-rule if I felt it best to break it. Last night it didn't feel best to break it.

"Do you know what was happening last night at the noodle bar? There was a small flock."

She best give me the gossip of what exactly was going on. As a best friend who always meandered around the farms finding new gossip and information, I was relying on her to tell me.

"You are right, there was a gathering. Why, were you there? I thought you guys would just go to the pub."

Well, that was a stupid thing to say. My plan to go to the pub was trampled on when Justin said he wanted a sturdy meal in his belly.

"I wanted to go to the pub, but Justin felt weak and wanted food. I suggested we went to the noodle bar on the high street."

I gained a nod from Charlene so didn't go into specifics about the kiss at the end of the night although I wanted to. At that moment when he pulled away, I believe it was the best kiss of my life. Far better than any kiss that was offered by Claude.

"So, you saw the group in the restaurant? See any faces that you recognised?"

Charlene was being completely ignorant of the large meeting or she was entirely knowledgeable of, the reasoning of the booking.

"Yes, I saw a couple of faces, but I don't know their names."

This was the part of the conversation where Charlene gives a lot of self-praise.

"Oh, that was annoying for you. I knew the group and who was going. It was a birthday meal and I know you're aware of the birthday boy. I'm surprised you didn't notice him!"

I did notice Richard, but I wanted to put him out of my mind and focussed on my date with Justin. I should react shocked and worthy of her knowledge. Charlene could have come along to hunt where the best place to sit with a decent view of Richard.

"Wow! That's great! I knew you'd know about the group. So, it was Richard's birthday you say? He looked like he was having a good time."

Charlene was quick to reply.

"He did, when I went over to his barn to wish him happy birthday from us, he told me he enjoyed the meal with his mates."

It was my turn to be open-mouthed. She did what? Did she actually go away to speak with my gorgeous crush without me? I sincerely hoped she had arranged for another meeting. My stomachs were behaving themselves nicely so I wouldn't have a problem with the food expulsion now.

The sudden uprightness occurred, and I knew something relatively important was going to be said by Charlene.

"He mentioned you were sat in the restaurant too."

Oh crap, I hoped I looked good for him. The light was pretty dull where I was sitting. This could have painted me as a goth, or a secret murderer. Both were unpleasing options to hold.

"I arranged for us to have a cooking teaching session with Justin."

"Have you arranged for this with Justin? He might be busy today."

The ball has been smashed in her side of the court. Hopefully he wouldn't be able to come.

"Yes, Justin is free to come. He'll be around my barn at six. By then, Barry would have prepared most of the technical examples."

So, this will be a case of forced fun. I've been told to stand by Barry and see how he cooks whilst showing an element of amazement and smiles. It was slightly interesting to be fair and I trotted off with the plan how best to make sweet potato chips.

'Hey, Justin! Long-time no-see!' Would be the first words I will say to him. I reckon he'd be a touch nervous as he seems a sensitive ram. I started to feel a flush of excitement to see him again. Charlene started to mess with my hair. She was probably trying to make Justin fall in love with me. I told her to stop when I heard the barn doors ring.

Charlene squealed as she rushed to the barn door. I questioned myself as to why she was so happy to receive a guest, who was my date from last night. Did she actually want to ask him why he kissed me or something?

"Oh, hi! We've just mentioned something about you at your dinner meal. She'd be excited to see you again! Stay here and I'll get her to see you."

A grumble grew louder and louder. Richard laid his hand on Charlene's shoulder and told her not to go up.

"Don't tell Shirley I'm here, I just wanted to talk to you actually."

Charlene started to gently stamp her hooves, something she does when she's excited.

"What would you like to talk to me about? Anything I can help you with?"

The grumble returned. After a couple of seconds, it ceased, and Richard waved goodbye as he left the barn.

Multiple leaps were had as Charlene came into her barn. I could instantly see she held some exciting news as her hands were flapping so quickly it was as if she wanted to fly. When the flapping slowed down to a near stop, she looked directly at me and said, "Richard."

It seemed only fair I should join in with the hand flapping. I asked questions to discover why she mentioned that name. Charlene must have felt she was grubby as I heard her switch on the shower. Maybe Richard was the one at the door. That would warrant the reason why she said his name when she got back to the living room. Yes. That must be the reason. She was out there for a good few minutes, four or maybe five at a push.

The barn door rang again. I didn't have any problem with leaping towards the door to be met with my farm crush.

"Hey, Shirley, I was actually speaking with your good friend just now. How are you?"

Justin seemed nicer looking than he was last night. He wasn't as good looking as Richard is in my opinion. My moral duty pushed me to give him an answer. I don't look as good as last night because of my lack of make-up but could smile broadly as a replacement.

"I'm very well, thank you, Justin. How are you?"

He then grabbed me and gave me a kiss. It was exactly as good as how I remembered it to be. That memory was soaked in red wine too. I heard trotters coming from my right and I sharply remembered Charlene being in the area sat in the living room. I pulled Justin to walk with me so we could sit in the living room.

Once sat, Charlene entered the room wrapped in a towel.

"Thanks for warming up the shower, Charl, I'll be two minutes. See you in a bit!"

Charlene made an eyeroll at me which I personally felt was rude as normally I do the same to her.

Once I was squeaky clean, I moved on to think about what topics of conversation the three were having when I was away. My self-interest told me it must include something to do with me. What if it wasn't? I needed to rush so I'm included.

"But wouldn't bake well?"

That was Justin's voice talking about something different to talking about me.

"My boyfriend, Barry, would be the one who answer questions relating to baking. Have you heard of the word, 'Aquafarba'?"

Justin really looked as if he was a new-born baby lamb. He shook his head in disagreement. I wanted to cuddle this ram to make him realise it's all right not to know.

Barry stamped in to the room and smiled broadly. You could sense he means business. Introductions aren't really my thing, so Charlene stepped in and said,

"This is Justin! Apparently, Shirley gave him a good answer to the P question."

Barry reached across to shake Justin's hand. He smiled and looked me directly in the eye.

"So, Shirley answered your protein question yes? She's a good ewe, she has been told about the sun giving us energy in green food."

I think she's a wise one Justin.

Chapter 17

It must have been past three before until we were all able to sit down in the living room. Barry displayed the reasons given to him as the vegan wonder ram. With each ingredient we were advised to put in our cooking bowls, Barry enlightened us about its history. Turmeric, for example, grew a sense of power by the Aztecs and its power of healing grew around the world because of its healing cure abilities.

"You should have a teaspoon of turmeric every day."

Barry gave us a knowing smile after saying that. That was enough to believe every word he was going to say going forward.

"I think I actually have a jar of turmeric in my cupboard, so I can use that going forward."

I thought it best to say something to give me extra points, not that the cooking afternoon was going to be a competition or anything like that. I am still quite the swat when it came to different subjects at school. When I bothered to turn up that is. Thankfully, Barry agreed with my nerd-based thinking when he said,

"Absolutely! Turmeric is a spice that's in many cupboards but most do not know how best to use it. That's why I want to get you guys knowing how."

I nodded my best to show I passionately concurred. Justin started to reach across the table to get a fingertip of turmeric. When he sat back down and sucked his finger covered in turmeric, he looked confused.

"It has a weird taste. You're saying we should have a bit of it each day?"

Barry was soon to answer.

"Well, you don't have to eat it directly from the jar. You could mask the 'weird' flavour by putting it into a tea or even better in a curry or hot meal. The options are endless."

He was magnetic with his talking and smile. I almost became jealous of Charlene, but I stopped myself when I thought about him taking away the time, she normally is with me. I should be thankful in a way. I couldn't hold sensible conversations with him like Charlene does, who really knows about countries? I'll focus my attention on something else.

Justin tilted his head slightly and sat down. It was a relief that he wouldn't say anything else. Oh no, he leant forward.

"The thing about this vegan thing, if I signed up to it, I'd just want to eat cheese."

I smiled at that comment because I went through the same thinking when I started being a vegan. Barry would probably have the best sentence to answer him. I hoped he would because I would come across as uneducated on that matter by just saying, "You can't break the vegan rules!"

"It's funny you should say that Justin because most think the same. The big dairy companies are actually very sneaky because they inject something into each cheese product. This is casein. It makes you want more of it after you've finished eating the cheese. What's even scarier is that Casein is everywhere, like everywhere. Food flavourings and protein bars and anything that has 'lactic acid' probably includes Casein. Beware that 'dairy-free' might have casein."

Justin genuinely looked shocked. I felt an urge to give him a cuddle to make him feel a sense of unity on this matter. When his mouth remained aghast for another minute, I decided to sweep in next to him for a cuddle.

"Okay, I reckon I could do no dairy. That's not a problem. I drink my coffee black anyway."

Barry pushed forward to be nearer Justin and told him about the number of products that have dairy in them. Cakes are a no-go area to eat. Ice Cream should be shunned as best as possible. Sorbets will have to do. I could sense that Justin wasn't as clear as how his nodding demonstrated. I thought it best to offer him some encouragement.

Without any sense of sound, Justin suddenly screamed out.

"EGGS!"

Barry smiled and raised his eyebrows. I knew exactly what he was going to say as I too have challenged Barry on this.

"Your friend, Shirley, asked me about this very same topic when she started veganism so I'll keep my answer as short as I can."

This will be a supreme answer and usurp my answer "it comes from a chicken's bottom."

To add a sense of importance, Barry linked his hands and raised them into the air to perform a stretch.

"Okay, Justin, this is a big subject so ask me any of your questions when they come up?"

Just like how he has previously done since being here, Justin confidently nodded at Barry. I looked across at Charlene and gained her attention. I waved to the door and held a questioning face. Thankfully, she smiled and nodded, got up to walk towards the door. I joined her at the front door when I heard the words "eggs are made of fat". These words made me decide that I wouldn't eat eggs again in my life.

Once we were both out of earshot the nattering could begin. The summary of our conversation was that I still really fancied Richard, Justin was a good kisser and I didn't really know what to do. Charlene giggled and grabbed my forearm.

"You and Justin look really good together you know?"

I wasn't entirely sure of what exactly she meant. Was she giving us a blessing or something? Did she not want me to focus on Richard? Did she fancy Richard? The answer to this was easy as Richard was just perfection. She must fancy Richard. She could help me with another question, "When did she sleep with Barry?"

Tears and small jerking happened after I asked that question. This was not supposed to happen. I was hoping for two days as that would perfectly align with both me and Justin.

I put my hand on her back in the hope of quelling the crying. The question wasn't meant to provoke this.

"It's just we really love each other but we haven't got around to actually being intimate yet. I can't say anything because he is so busy all of the time. I don't even know if he is good, I've just made him out to be, he is excellent at whatever he tries. Trying to get gas guzzling lorry drivers to go vegan was a mammoth ask, but he did it."

I spun to look at her in the face.

"When we go back, hopefully Barry has told Justin about the court case against a dairy industry who published the line 'Eggs are healthy' and they lost the case as that couldn't be further from the truth. After he says that, you're going to have a passionate kiss with him."

Charlene screwed up her face and mumbled, "Okay."

We trotted up the hallway and disappeared into the living room. Just as expected, Barry said exactly the same as what he said to me.

I sat down opposite Justin and he smiled angelically back to me. This would be fun if he wanted to stay around.

A smile back, led on to me giving the best vegan fact that I think. My face was close to his, so I pecked him on the cheek.

"Honestly, babe, once you cut dairy you'll be as thin as a wafer. I'm serious, you'll drop the weight off."

My weight-loss insight was probably lost on Justin, he probably just runs around the fields in this area if he ever wanted to lose weight. He didn't have to because his figure looked quite satisfying when I had a chance to gain evidence. His legs aren't as long as Richard's, but they hold a sense of muscular shaping. I liked that.

Barry beckoned us all to the kitchen. Like soldiers on parade, we marched over to the kitchen. When Barry told us to weigh out the desired weighting of flower. We all took turns to do this and then were instructed to measure the recipe's desire of olive oil.

"This oil gets a bit slippery but is the best alternative to butter. Trust me, when we've finished, we'll have the best vegan brownies."

This was the point where I wondered if Charlene had tested Barry's brownies. She has told me she has tested lots of Barry's food creations, so she probably has.

When we had finished and started to pack up, I thought it best to sneak a few brownie pieces in my bag so I could eat some whilst watching evening television. That was if Justin didn't want to stay over. This was something that I thought he would want to do. We've kissed multiple times so it was evident that he would want to have nookie.

The final words from Barry were quite impressive. Definitely words I should remember going forward.

"There is no such word as 'can't' when it comes to veganism. Some say, 'I can't go vegan because I like cake too much', but veganism isn't about taking anything away, it's about gaining everything. Remember, there are always alternatives to whatever food you want to eat."

I yearned for Barry to tell Justin about the taste-buds flowering when you go vegan and the sensitivity to salt. My food order to the fast food restaurant could have been used as an example. I wouldn't be offended if he said that.

Starting up on my vegan diet again wasn't as difficult as the first time I started three weeks ago. So much has happened in such a relatively short piece of time. The most outstanding, being the fact that Charlene and Barry have not shared a mattress. This made it obvious to me as to why she got so excited when I told her about my love life. A wave of sympathy came over me for her.

My mattress was shared with Justin that night.

The next morning was a bit of a surprise, not only did I use my vocal chords to scream out to Justin about a topic, but I had the first rumblings of a crush growing. My tummy flickered when he brought me a cup of morning tea and another of his flashing good smile. Something I had mentioned to him before to make me feel confident around me. I coupled this with a light brushing of his wool and a grin.

The night was sensibly energetic and calm. Quite the opposite of the last sexual events I had with Claude, so it was enjoyable to get my breath back and feel the sensations of what was all around me. This joy was almost all blemished when he discovered that vegans weren't frail and weak.

I needed to say something that counteracts this.

"Oh, Justin you've fallen into the stereotypical belief. Vegans are definitely not weak, because they have a low body fat content, they find building muscle easier. You need to ask Barry about his friend, Rich. Apparently, he's done the most Ironman's on a vegan diet. If I wanted to be a weightlifter, I could. But I'd need to eat more food and I don't have time for that."

Justin just offered a weak laugh and looked the other way. The following silence was bearable and I didn't feel the need to speak. If I did, I would probably damage the sound work I've done offloading the science I said.

He came over to me and cupped my head in his hands. When he delivered one of his magical kisses, I felt the sexual tension rise between us. This was something I had briefly experienced with Claude on our first dates. It was magical to feel the same way again. It didn't take long before I considered if Richard would create the same response if I were to be in this situation.

Fed up of thinking about what ifs, I grabbed his hands and pulled him onto the mattress to resume what we had half an hour ago. The same enjoyment continued, and I didn't want this to end.

When it did, I did my complementary finger dancing around his body and kissed him on the cheek. He seemed to like that by his smiling. It was perfection. Everything didn't warrant a phone to interrupt us, but unfortunately it did.

Simultaneous groaning was shared between us. I thought whoever was the disruptor deserves a good eye roll and tuts. Justin's phone was the culprit which rang with the most awful theme tune. It most certainly wasn't upbeat and could even have a few random German words shouted to add to its craziness. Charlene's happy positive ringtone sounded like a magnificent symphony in comparison. I wondered who the caller was.

"Hi there, Jim! How you doing?"

Who the hell was Jim? No rams in my field are called Jim. I needed to pay attention even more. Thankfully, Justin has a high phone volume, so I could easily hear what the caller was saying. I moved my ear closer to his phone whilst the conversation continued. I couldn't decipher much which was frustrating.

After hearing Justin say "aha" over and over again he ended the call with, "See you in a bit," then hung up the phone. I did my best to show myself as puzzled for when he looked at me.

"Sorry, Shirley, I need to meet a mate. I'll try my best to come back but I can't make any promises."

After saying that, Justin rushed to get dressed and put his jacket on, as if he was on a sinking ship and needed to get out. "Bye then!" I shouted but didn't receive a reply.

My mind started whirring about what Justin was up to, who was this 'Jim' and why was he so desperate to get out? Was I really that bad between the sheets? Thinking too much on this matter will only solidify it as truth. I needed to think of something else, or better yet − ask Charlene about this Jim. She'd probably know of him. That's if she answered her phone. After hearing ringing for a minute, I gave up and went for a shower. Possibly the worst place to go if your mind is full of thoughts, each thought became exemplified and with no clear answer given, it became frustrating.

Patting myself dry and moisturising around my body I looked at my phone. My silent wishing finally turned out to be true, Charlene called me when I actually wanted her to. Normally, her ringing me tended to happen during inconvenient times like preparing to go to sleep, watching a movie when I wanted to see how the film ends and preparing a dinner that needs full attention. Now though, I was ready to have a full discussion with her. The main question I wanted answering was about this Jim.

"Hey, darling! Lovely to take your call!"

I always knew I needed to act super happy whenever I conversed with her because to not do so would make me sound really dull and slightly depressed. Charlene would be keen to be the first to sort out and help me in any way. The top of her skills was the farm gossip of this area, so I best test her knowledge.

"Hi, Shirl, your advice worked wonders for me!"

Those were words I'd never believed to hear. What was she going on about? The tip regarding the best hand motion to moisturise the face?

"From you suggesting I should passionately kiss Barry, led to us both sharing the same mattress and doing stuff."

I didn't need the cheesy eyebrow raising and wink to tell me they finally had sex. I just tilted my head slightly and said, "Awe." This was a pointless head movement as I was speaking on the phone. It felt good doing it and I really wanted to get into the heart of to speak with my mission to find out who this ram was who interrupted mine and Justin's snuggle time. Who was he?

"We stayed in bed for a long time. We are probably going to do the same again tonight!"

It seemed a good enough time to start my questioning. I'm glad that my order to Charlene worked out well, in fact perfectly, but I needed to know about this 'Jim'. I had a dreadful feeling it will end up badly regarding Justin. Like he was a drug dealer and was wanting to use innocent Justin in some awful way. My flag was flying to protect him in whatever way I can. My eyes looked over at Charlene to deliver me the fate regarding Jim.

"Oh Jim? He's cool, knows quite a lot of sheep in these areas. Not as many as me I might add. Why have you asked me about Jim? It's quite an odd question to ask because we've never spoken about him before."

Learning the fact that Jim exists and isn't a ghost and actually exists puts my mind at rest. It does, however, make me wonder why Justin was in such a rush to go out to meet him. My mind began to whir again, the same way as when I took a shower.

"Why would Justin want so desperately want to see him?"

My volume inadvertently started to rise when saying that. I hoped that question would be answered quickly by the self-called gossip queen.

"Well, Justin is an old mate of Jim. He even went out with one of Jim's daughters. Yes, I remember."

My volume suddenly exploded when I said, "YOU KNEW THAT AND DIDN'T TELL ME?"

I instantly felt sorry for shouting that. I didn't want to ruin any of Charlene's post coital bliss, but this was something I really wanted to know. Annoyance was the biggest feeling swirling around in my past mind. Why did she not mention this to me when she knew I was preparing myself for a date with Justin? A simple message of her knowledge of his ex-girlfriend wouldn't have gone amiss.

"Ah babe, I'm sorry. I just didn't really want to get involved. You might have forced me to do more clothes buying and do more make-up on you. That would have made you look terrible. You went on the date looking incredible. It's his loss if he wanted to leave you to see an old ram."

That gave me a slight boost. Just needed to put the matter to the back of my mind. I could, of course, send Justin a message enquiring why he disappeared from my bedroom all of a sudden and more importantly how he is going to pay me back from the sudden amount of stress and confusing behaviour. I was hoping it was a holiday or clothes shopping. Those two things could be taken as atonement from him. Maybe a nice car could be thrown in too, it really was an awful spot to be in when his trotter sound fell silent and he left me alone.

Out of interest, I grabbed my phone to check it was still empty of messages. It was, so I placed it back on the table in a place where I could easily grab it if I had any communication at all. I decided to watch a film that I had, one where I've never got to watch until the end. It was at this time when I thought it would be good to have Justin sat next to me. Whatever he's doing I'd do anything to get him back and giving me those wonderful kisses again.

I decided to ring him. Surely, he would answer me and give me a short message of what he was up to? When the ringing lasted for a minute, I decided to give up. It clicked with me that I had rung Charlene earlier in the same way. She was possibly more bothered by having sex instead of answering my call.

I really hoped Justin wasn't doing the same.

Chapter 18

The first day back at work was timed for a torrent of rainfall.

I didn't expect the farmer to call off work, we were lucky to have a day off back in winter, so the shots of water droplets were bearable if I were to be paid. Charlene could make the day better if she was to deliver me news regarding Justin and his whereabouts. My mind still hasn't stopped working on it.

So, this old ram has signed off one of his daughters as a girlfriend for Justin. That was my deduction of it. I could be wrong, but in my mind, Justin and his ex-girlfriend were happily walking down the high street together. I have no idea of what she looks like. She must be good looking to go out with Justin as he is very good looking too.

Charlene came closer to me and held a grave face. She kind of got me worried about Justin's health.

I grabbed her by the shoulder and asked her very calmly and clearly for my standards, "What's wrong?"

Charlene just nodded which was enormously aggravating. I rewarded myself for staying calm and not displaying any screaming that was happening in my mind. Thankfully, Charlene decided to speak

"Hey babe, I only just found out about Jim and what exactly is going on with Justin and the full case. I know you've only just started work but do you want to take a break?"

The grass had been grazed enough over the weekend's extra work I had put in. Extra free time should have been for R&R but I just wanted to get out and do something and maybe make the farmer notice.

"Sure, I'm free! Let's go get a coffee to discuss this Justin news. Let's go!"

The pair of us scampered out of the field in the opposite direction of the grazing workers were going. When we dashed into a coffee shop and sat, we both sighed. I looked directly at Charlene in the eyes to employ her to speak.

"I'm going to get coffees for us to drink, are you all right with coconut lattes? Or do you want almond?"

It was difficult to not feel annoyance. She was after all buying the coffees for our promptly set up meeting. What I would have preferred was for her to ditch the caffeinated buying experience and come and sit down opposite me to relay the news she had found out about both Jim and Justin.

Once she had returned, I thanked her and leaned in. This felt like a top-secret meeting.

"So, what have you found and most importantly is Justin alive? He hasn't been answering any of my calls or texts."

I didn't appreciate her cackling through laughter. She could have just told me he was alive and well, she was of course the queen of gossip, but I wished she could use tact sometimes.

"Justin is alive and well, but he is busy at the moment something that doesn't involve you and you're not the cause of."

I took a large slurp of the coffee in front of me. It was a surprise I wasn't the cause of anything as that counters most of the things that happens with my life anyway. I had a feeling she didn't want to continue for much more of the topic. So, I felt it was my duty to press her for more information.

"What is it that he's doing? Why am I not involved? I did have his dick in me the other night, remember?"

Charlene instantly sparked up to say, "You did use a condom right?!"

She sounded scarily alarmed. I panicked if she knew Justin had a STI or some sort of contagious disease. She probably would know this sort of thing as she knows all the gossip that's around the place so I wouldn't put it past her to know of the medical records too.

I calmed her down by saying, "Of course, Justin had a johnnie on. You know I only have sex if the ram puts a helmet on his soldier. You know that!"

Instant relaxation filled the coffee shop. Her words still haven't given me too much information on why he was busy and was it to do with Jim? Did they have a fight? That would fit what she initially said regarding me not being involved.

"Okay, that's cool then. I didn't want you to get involved with a baby or anything."

A gleaming smile was given to her, similar to the ones I gave her boyfriend when he was teaching us about food.

"I only say that because Justin has become a father with his ex, who's Jim's daughter."

I didn't believe that to be true. The ram who I shouted "bye" seemed highly sensible and one who wouldn't want a baby. No, Charlene must have got it wrong.

Working was full of unanswerable questions.

"Who was this ex? The baby must be adorable because of the genetics of the parents. That's if Justin found her attractive. Why does everyone need to have babies before me? Utterly selfish in my opinion."

Charlene did her new best-friend duty and nodded whilst I was speaking.

"Do you want to go and see this baby?"

Charlene rarely silences me, but the question was intriguing. Do I really want to go and see another baby if I don't have to? If I went, I'd probably come into contact with Justin, but I didn't want to do that. Over the past couple of days since we met on our date, I heard things weren't perfect between us. I dissuaded myself from holding any romantic feelings for him.

This was a tactic I used with Claude my ex heart-breaking boyfriend, but it didn't stop me from having an unplanned night together. The opposite of what I was wanting.

"She's in Burley hospital birthing unit. Apparently, they have a water birthing available there. We should go! We won't be in anyone's trouble and it would be a good trip out of here."

No happiness was felt by me with that invitation. It seemed stupid. Both of us did not want to have a baby. It would just end up being a day trip from hell. I heard the howling mothers giving birth to their lambs whilst I was visiting my cousin who had a bad fall once and was forced to go to hospital. I will never forget the sounds of pain emitted.

"I wouldn't mind taking a look, actually."

Why on earth would Charlene want to take a look where the most painful experience happens in an ewe's life? It would be a sick form of voyeurism in my opinion. We were settled on not having any lambs for now. Before we left for a night out, we'd check if we had a rubber, Charlene used her bra as the best holder for such an item.

"No. No, Charlene."

A definitive tone was set, and I didn't expect a challenging answer. Or anything other than an "okay". It was a mild shock when I heard her speak again.

"Please, Shirley? I know it's been recent coupling between me and Barry, but I think we'll be planning on looking into the lamb side of things between us."

Wow. No. I've had a day full of shocks. Firstly, my new ram of my town and then my kind of best friend thinking of having a lamb. The action of which must result in using the name Shirley in some way. It would be rude not to.

"Umm, okay sure. But I do want Barry to cook me one of his delicious meals. If you are capable of doing that for me then of course, I'll come."

Cue the yippees and squealing. The giggle and full hug was made by Charlene.

"I will do my best on the Barry cheffing front, but I think he would love to do that for you. In fact, I'm certain of it."

My arm was grabbed and walked to the front gates of the farm. It didn't take long to trot along to Burley. My dictation for the journey was Charlene giving me vegan health facts for rams.

Apparently, they last for thirty percent longer until they squish, when they eat a vegan diet. This was something Barry was proud of and he spread this fact around to other rams.

Almost immediately after stepping a hoof in the delivery department, the screams shocked our ear drums. Having had past experience of this when my cousin was in hospital, I could easily prepare for this situation. Charlene on the other hoof looked utterly scared. I wanted to smile at her to make things all right.

After wandering around the curtained beds and hearing the screams of agony, I thought it was best to direct Charlene by the arm to the exit.

"Why were there so many tiny bottles on the shelves? Didn't see any tea urns around the hospital to use them with."

Charlene had a sudden movement to attention. I was familiar with this, either she would deliver something spectacular or it would just be verbal rubbish.

"The tiny bottles were filled with human breast milk. Barry told me about this. The mother is the best source of milk. Stealing milk from another animal messes up the system. After all we're sheep, not cows. To think otherwise would set the path to get to really bad diseases. Like really bad autoimmune diseases."

I needed to quieten her down in some way. She was sounding too smart in front of me. There was a seldom sheep trotting to the delivery unit entrance. Within seconds apart, Charlene let out a quiet squeal.

"Justin!"

Oh dear, how was I to play this? Heartbroken damsel, left by herself to build her ego after being left without a goodbye?

I didn't have to try too hard with appearance as Justin just mouthed the word "Sorry" and passed me.

Chapter 19

My moral compass urged me not to be too severe upon my new best friend, Charlene, but I felt I needed to say something to demonstrate my opinion on the matter. I agreed with what she was saying, but her cheerful demeanour was arguing with what we could easily have for breakfast and drink in our coffees. Having the option to drink the other milks was cool, coconut lattes were on my coffee ordering list because it made me feel I was on holiday when I drank it. Charlene assured me that non-dairy milks didn't go off, so I didn't have to rush to keep the milk bottles in their cool fridge home all of the time.

I had to give it to her, Charlene was really standing by her man on the cow milk front. When she told me about the oddity of drinking milk made by a mother of a completely different species to my own, I felt terrible.

I was urged to turn back to the hospital to speak with Justin. That was a no.

"No, Charlene, I am definitely not going to do that. If Justin really wanted to say something to me then he can walk back out to where we're standing. No."

Her low volume groaning started. This was something she had done repeatedly throughout the time we had been friends. I'd never had been so annoyed since now. Why did Charlene feel so strongly about me making friends with Justin? What service could it provide for her? I was settled in not doing anything romantic with Justin. Something I thought she knew from my continuous blasting of his character since he walked out to do parent things. Yes, I definitely said bad things about Justin implying that I did not fancy him anymore. My heart directorate was now on Richard. It was now difficult to achieve this.

Whilst I was thinking about the direction my heart should go regarding Richard, I noticed Charlene darting off to enter the hospital again. She must have really enjoyed looking at the lambs.

I followed her as that was what a new best friend does, and I was surprised to find her talking with Justin. The menacing escapee. What were they talking about? If it was I then I hoped I came off best with a dazzling review.

"Yeah I saw them yesterday. William was most proud to be a godparent."

Oh. They were talking about William. The devil cupid who set me up with Justin. Looking back to the tea rooms where my date was concocted with the gay couple who was in overwhelming love, it seemed too good to be true they could suggest a ram of my dreams. Justin was a good attempt, but they overlooked the fact that he was a father and was possibly not a ram looking for love.

I moved closer to the couple talking. They both held serious faces.

"Shirley? How are you doing babe? Sorry I left your place after staying with you. I just needed to leave for a personal reason."

My mouth didn't hold any sense of delay when I spoke.

"Personal, like what? Seeing your new lamb being delivered? I found out about this and I really didn't believe it to be true. It is true now and I'll take a few trots backwards to give you some free time."

Justin gasped when I said that. The silent treatment was given. With a big hard stare to emphasise the situation's severity. He used my internal goods as a pleasurable Willy hugger. Then scampered as if I was a disease-ridden pest. Which was hurtful. Claude came into my memory at this moment, as he performed similar scampering trick. Maybe I should consider myself to be the causer of the boyfriend offender.

"Look, Shirley, I had a wonderful date with you and the selection of restaurant was truly wonderful. Our night we shared was magic, learning things from Barry and then give being with you was truly fantastic. Your kiss makes my spine shiver and I'm truly gutted things have turned out this way. Please, forgive me?"

Well, that was a charming delivery. The best part being he really enjoyed my kisses. It was great to know I felt the same about his kiss.

What an option to be left with, should I forgive him? My gut told me no. This was a shame as I really enjoyed spending time with him. Charlene worked her slam down vocals by saying, "You have really hurt Shirley and if she has any sense, she would run as far away from you as possible. You are a womaniser, Mr Justin and I can't believe I spent so much time on her ensemble and make-up for your date together."

I was impressed, when Charlene wanted to be mean she really knew how to pull the vocabulary trigger. I sensed it was best to leave the Justin stage after she said that.

As we walked arm in arm down the high-street, I gained a sense of wellbeing, I wasn't decided by Justin and I could look forward for pastures anew with hopefully a new ram that I can live happily ever after. Ideally this ram's name starts with the letter R.

"You're better than that, Shirl, he was just a lucky ram that you were set up with. Set up really badly. Who did you say set you up with Justin? They should be shunned anytime you meet them."

Sorry, my tea drinking gentle ram but I'm about to turn you in.

"Actually, it was a couple who you've met. I went to the tea shop with William and Steve and asked if they could set me up on a date. So, they did, with Justin. You cannot blame them for any heart bruising they did. Maybe they weren't aware of Justin being a dad."

Charlene let out a *pfft* sound. She shook her head and hunted for her phone in her bag. When she held it in her palm, she raised a finger up at me.

"I'm just going to call William to sort out what exactly went wrong with his cupid's bow."

I enjoyed that sentence, something obviously went wrong on the date planning debauchery. I wouldn't mind having a glass of wine in the pub to recall exactly what went wrong. Yes, that's the plan, hopefully tonight.

"Hi, William! How are you doing Mr? Yes, yes…I know! Yes. Absolutely! Yes, all right. Pub later? I have Shirley with me, and I'm sure has questions about why you thought Justin was the best date for her. Utterly rubbish dude, I'm afraid. What now?"

Charlene pulled her mouth away from the handset and asked me if I wanted to speak with William. I did, of course, but none were happy and thankful. She passed the phone on to me.

"William? Yes, I'm very well, thanks. What the devil were you on setting me up with Justin? Yes, he is good look-ing, but he is also unattainable. He was soon to be a father. Were you not aware of this fact?"

William seemed highly flustered when he answered my questions. Apparently, Justin was newly single, and William and Steve thought we were a genuine good match. Credit was bestowed upon them for that. We did have a good date. I reckon Steve had a thing for him though, just a sense after warning me about Justin not looking as good as he was. A blatant challenge for his affections, it doesn't matter now though. Both of my cupids should have given the down-low of his ex-girlfriend and mother of his child.

"He didn't fully answer my questions, but he did apolo-gise. He didn't expect Justin would act in the same way as he did to me."

My eyes looked to Charlene and we both shrugged. My quest to find love with Richard continues. Charlene sensed my thought patterns and told me some strengthening romance words.

"You will find someone good, Shirley, I can just sense it. It may not be the ram you want most but the special one will probably be hidden around the corner. Just you continue do-ing what you do, and your dream ram will just appear."

What is Charlene talking about? Does she really think she's some sort of mystic? What has she been eating? I know Barry really adores mushrooms, but she must have had a special batch of mushrooms by the way she's going on. I thanked her and said, "I hope so."

Bizarrely, Charlene let out a scream. She was holding her phone and looking at it whilst smiling. I never get as excited as she does but I am inquisitive about the matter.

"Oh my god! Barry is going to be on television! His idea for a healthy living show has just been commissioned by one of the major broadcasters! He's been wanting to do it for ages and now it's finally come true!"

That's great news, but my mind soon switched to celebratory drinks in the pub and wondering if I would ever meet someone famous from TV land if Barry was going to be working there.

"That's great news, pass on my support to Barry when you next see him? Also, tell him that I'd be happy to be a production assistant if he would ever want one."

I once heard about someone making it big from just asking for a measly job on set once. With Barry being signed to do a big show then it wouldn't cause any harm in asking for a job. I might brush my shoulders among a heartthrob that's on the biggest soap at the moment.

Charlene giggled and told me she definitely would let Barry know about my inquisitiveness regarding the shooting.

"I'm not too sure what it will look like, it may even be shot in my kitchen at home!"

Well, that's not exciting. I've been there plenty of times.

Chapter 20

The sun rise came beaming through the bedroom windows at a stupid morning hour. It made me think about when the time changes to a more acceptable time like how everyone else wakes up. My morning sunrise alarm clock needed to be functional at a later time, this will coincide when the majority of the farm wakes up.

The cows were awake as I could hear the gentle moos that were rolling down the hill side. I rolled over and pushed my curtain sash to the side, so I would have a better view of the farm. I had obviously just seen a birth as the mother cow was nursing her calf and licking its head. Very endearing to look at and was probably just like how I looked like as a baby lamb. Obviously, I was cuter than a smelly calf. I watched the silhouette of mother cow bend its head to the blob she was licking all over. I decided to attack the next task of the morning; breakfast needed preparing. I rolled down my duvet in readiness to get out of the bed. I glanced outside to my viewing I was previously looking at. A massive SUV rolled up the steep hill to an abrupt stop near to the cow and the calf. Two humans circled near to the calf and then suddenly body slammed the poor baby cow and shoved it into the SUV the cow stomped her hoofs and followed the calf. She bellowed out so loud that it could be heard from where I was sat in my farm. The two humans must have been vets as they quickly handled and took the baby calf away from its mum. Something nobody wants to happen. I hope the calf gets better and is reunited with mum. He probably will do as I don't think the farmer would do anything as mean as that.

My phone buzzed, time for Charlene to give me the local gossip.

"Justin's ex-girlfriend had anaemia and it was a surprise to them both that she became pregnant. They had previously been apart for around three months, so no wonder Will and Steve set you guys up. It was completely unexpected she would become holding a bun in the oven. Oh, and that thing you said about Steve liking Justin? Bang on – well done. I didn't notice that when I last saw Steve. I think you're going to take my crown as Gossip Queen with that subtle observation. I doth my cap to you."

That daily Charlene chat was worth the amount of time I used to listen to her. The pregnant woman was anaemic. I thought that was when you had white hair and blue eyes. That was something I needed to find out about before I left to start work. There were forty minutes before I actually had to step out of my barn to travel to work. Plenty of time to open my laptop and log on to the internet. If scandalous gossip suddenly appeared on my screen I wouldn't have been offended.

I thanked Mr Google for helping me spell anaemia. He even read my mind as when I started my search it immediately came up with a search term, 'Anaemia in pregnancy'.

I really didn't want it to happen, but I had a flicker of sympathy for Justin's ex. It sounded like a trial to manage whilst pregnant.

A spell of clarity and clear thinking came over me. No wonder Justin was so desperate to leave me and get to the maternity ward. His kind heart must have been worried about his ex. I'm aware they had broken up, but the foundation of the relationship would still exist. In many ways like me and Claude. Except for the unplanned rampant intercourse session.

Once it got down to ten minutes before work started, I collected all of my belongings that aided me throughout the day and said goodbye to my mirror. When I reached my front door, I could hear the screaming made by the mother cow I'd watched earlier. I hoped they had healed the baby cow that they had taken away. Hopefully, by the time I get home from work.

"Shirley! Come here! Chloe has broken up with Claude and has been chucking out all of his stuff he left in her bedroom! Things are all over the place, one ram picked up one of Claude's black sunglasses!"

This is the kind of news I liked, something had a personal motive for me. I wish I had done something like this to him before. Maybe when he spent the night away from home the third time. I wanted to give that ewe Chloe a high-five.

"Babe, I don't want to freak you out or anything but there is a sheep coming towards us. A sheep who you have declared fancying."

Oh my, Richard must be coming. I haven't even had time to do my second coating of make-up. This is terrible, breathing in and out calmly is the only way I could do this meet.

"Oh no, wait, Shirl. It's not your biggest crush that's walking towards us – it's who I've just mentioned."

It would have been Justin who she means. My heart could relax after dancing around franticly thinking it was going to be Richard who would be the ram I was going to meet. Suddenly, it was Justin standing in front of me. And his face must have gone through expert make-up being applied as he looked more gorgeous than when we had our date. Quite remarkable, I didn't notice just how good looking he really was.

"Hey, Shirley, how are you?"

Should I say something really cutting, referencing my lonely stay at home by myself after he ran out? Or should I leave it being relaxed and cool? I didn't want him to feel I thought his actions were acceptable. Of course, now I know exactly what the reasons were to prompt such a dramatic exit from my bedroom. That doesn't mean I've forgiven him for it. I wonder how he is going to play things.

"I'm good. Thanks, Justin."

Played it impartial, but cool. I even offered a smile to finish the sentence off. He didn't take too long to reply, a meaningless tactic that degrades anything he was going to say next.

115

"I just really fancied getting away somewhere ideally with a beach and a swimming pool. I'm not the best solo traveller so after the time we had together, I just wanted to know if you wanted to come with me?"

Now I needed to discuss something like this with Charlene. She was stood on the far side of the field. Typical. My wide grin would act as a pause whilst I reached Charlene to tell her this exciting question and ask her what I should do. If he was going to pay for me to come with him to whatever dream world he had just described, I would say yes in a heartbeat. I've come to learn that Charlene had the best knowledge for when it comes to most decisions. It was slightly gutting when I wanted to get a tattoo and she told me not to go anywhere near the tattoo parlour as I would just regret it. Annoyingly, she probably served to be right. Listening to the tattoo machines just sent a chill down my spine.

I awaited what she thought of my good holiday offer.

"Charlene, Justin has just asked me if I'd go on a holiday with him to a place where there's a beach and is nice and warm. He didn't mention it but there would probably be cocktails too."

Her response didn't have to begin with a big sigh. It made her response start negatively. My hope was for her to be really positive without the accusing stance that she'd adopted. Okay, she's going to shut down what could be the holiday of my life which will all be paid for.

"Shirley, I love you. I know, you know, but what Justin has offered you is nothing more than a dream. You may want to believe it is true and there might actually be a real spot on the globe but really? We have only just said about him being a new dad. This is probably something he would enjoy being. He is a good ram, everyone can't say a bad word about him but do you want to take time away from him being a good dad? If you go, you will have a good time but always feel something dragging you in your stomachs. Do you love Justin?"

That was a stark question from her that I didn't expect. Do I love Justin? That got me thinking. I did like him enormously, but the big L word was still quite far away for me. So, in some way I did but in other ways I didn't. This led me into a predicament. I should hurry back if I really loved him. I needed to trot to him and ask for some more information. Before I darted back, Charlene gave me a question to see if I loved Justin.

"Okay, so the barns are all on fire."

A quizzical furrowed brow was given by me.

"Just imagine this to be true. There are flames all around, but someone hands you a phone to make your last call. Who are you going to call? And don't say 'Fire brigade'. You could really find out who loves if you do this test."

That was such a clever question and I needed to think about who my last call would be. I thought about it all the way to the other side of the field. I couldn't see Justin where I last left him when I trotted over to Charlene, to check on my new holiday dilemma. Like a magician, he had just disappeared, although he was stood chatting to an unknown ewe. She was smiling and nodding. Then it clicked with me that he gave the same dream holiday lines as he had given me. What a dick.

Chapter 21

This was a confusing day as it started off with a confusion. The moos coming from the farm opposite had increased its volume and just continued from when the vets had taken the calf away in their big van. I hope they'll bring it back soon though, as the mummy cow was continuing screaming out to it. The farmer must be aware of this and be sorting out getting the calf back from the cow hospital as no one would willing do that to their own cow. Especially when it was tame and loving like this cow was. The cow seemed to have been too depressed, happy to skip to the milking sheds so she couldn't have been too depressed. The sun rose at an earlier time than yesterday, I think, so I descended the stairs to the kitchen.

It was always easy being a non-vegan as you could eat whatever you wanted for breakfast. I could do with a large Danish with a cherry on top. My mouth began to salivate just thinking about it. Charlene's words nee Barry would start to repeat themselves by saying, "You can always find an alternative," and it felt like the toy versions of them in my head stood with their hands out, shaking their fingers at me. If I were a non-vegan then I would trot off to the bakery and dance down the aisles and maybe even take a bite out of one of the cakes that were on display, wiping the cream from my lips. I would be happy then. Unless, I took a moment to actually think about how many of my farm friends' family members were used and killed to produce a food item that acted so friendly in my mouth. There will be no slaughter, cutting or physically punishing to innocent animals if I stick with my vegan diet. At this point, my mini toy versions of Charlene and Barry danced around in my mind shouting, 'Yipee!!!' I felt secure in my thinking that veganism is the right thing to do.

My phone vibrated on the table, it was time to find out what the gossip was around these areas by answering Charlene's call.

"Hi babe, how are you?"

I sat down and arranged myself to be comfortable. This usually lasts longer than two minutes if it really was a briefing.

"I'm really well, thanks. Are you sat down because I have big news to tell you!"

That raised my eye line, but I always held the notion of doubt in my mind whenever she starts with an opening sentence like that.

"Go on, I'm listening."

The loud cow screaming really needed to stop and give the poor calf back to its mother. Charlene's voice was quite loud, so I could hear her over the racket of the fuss and all of the screaming that was coming from the mother cow.

"Good, okay that date that we prepared yourself for Justin was all a worthless to get you into bed with him. Yes, it was. I went over to find where William is, after I spoke with you and he started by saying that he didn't mean to upset you and he didn't know Justin's ex was pregnant."

Well, I knew both of them were sorry for the worst date set-up but was that all she was going to say?

"That's not all I'm going to say; it turns out that Justin is an ewe ram. He used to go out with countless ewes before he moved here. He was even trying it on with new-ewe, Rachel, yesterday. After we spoke, I looked across the field and could see them energetically chatting."

I felt the need to show my concurrence.

"Yes, I saw that! I walked over to where I saw him last in order to offer my answer to his question. I am so glad you told me not to go with him. He was probably lying about that and if we ended up going, he'd just be eyeing up the new ewes that would be trotting around. They probably be flouncing their bodies and wearing thongs and sparkling bikini tops. Of which I don't own and if I did, wouldn't wear them outside. Especially not anywhere exciting like the beach or seaside."

Charlene excitedly nodded. And smiled at me. Thinking about it, my romance attraction has hit a bump in the love journey road. My destination is still clear; the vegan hunk Richard.

"I'm glad you saw that! I'm pretty sure that didn't upset you too much. We said goodbye to him and now it's on to a new ram. Yes, I know your over the top with Richard, so you don't have to let me know on that front!"

Having a wing-ewe could prove vital on this task which I have code named 'Operation V' as he was the reason I wanted to turn vegan. Since deciding, I have heard of countless of other reasons. All of them I agree with. All of them, except one. It is not vegan to wear wool. That is complete codswallop, having a decent farm which treats my mates with respect it is totally fine to wear wool. I can remember Barbara from where I worked a few farms ago who didn't have a shearing for about a year. Granted that she was afraid of calories and walked around majestically even though she had piled on the weight from not eating the standard vegan diet, had made herself look like a fluffy white ball from not having a decent hair trim. My new waistline can fully agree with the notion regarding veganism as a weight-loss tool. Barry gets a bit mad when someone says this in front of him. He stripped me down when I mentioned this to him, I wanted to dive under the floorboards when he screamed things like, "IT IS NOT A WEIGHTLOSS TOOL!" he wanted to make it clear that although the sudden drop of eating no saturated fat of milk and butter does mean there's often weight loss.

"So, Ms farm gossip queen, when will be the next time he is around? If it's soon, do you fancy doing another walk down the high street to source any charity finds? Hopefully if we find something good, a date with Richard won't go down the pan as it has with Justin. Tsk."

Another happy series of squeaks came from Charlene enjoyed them. I similarly enjoyed listening when she was happy, but I was keen to hear her answer to my question.

"Umm, I think he's around this way now. Wait – what's the date? I've been told that's going out on pay day and that's usually the last working day of the month. So, this month it's the 28th. We've got two days before we make you look amazing for 'accidentally' bumping in to Richard. Sound like a plan?" My smile was fixed the moment she mentioned he was going out to somewhere around here. Days, so that will be one day for shopping and the other for make-up. Fate had walked in to say 'hello', by being the perfect date controller.

"Uh-oh, Charl, what if Justin disrupts our buying experience? He is a nice guy, but he could be a devil in disguise."

He was very emotive when he was with me but as a lover-ram he would be. Nevertheless, acknowledging that he could spring up unannounced was valid in mentioning the risks of Operation V.

"If we come across him just mouth the word 'BYE'. Just like what he did to you by pathetically mouthing the word 'sorry' when you saw him by the hospital. Just leave it. He might have wooed you to the bedroom but just remember how he left the bedroom. You're better than that and will likely woo Richard by yourself."

I thought her cheeky wink was justified so I neglected any eyerolling. My thoughts could turn towards anything beauty and ensemble related. A nice dress would certainly catch his attention. I jerked upright. That was the same mission I had with Justin. I needed another mission. I settled on getting a lovely skirt. Maybe a long, floaty one? That's quite alluring and would set me off well when I finally meet him.

The guy is like a legend. I might get tongue tied and nervous when I finally meet him. Charlene put my mind at ease when she spoke to me.

"Don't be a silly billy, when you guys finally meet it will just be wonderful. He will enjoy meeting you as he has previously said. Remember? He said he wanted to take you out for a drink. I'm sure he'll ignore vomit gate with the sea of vomit you created. Yes, I'm sure that the meet will work out perfectly. Honest!"

My trust with what she was saying was absolute. She normally gets these things right. My thinking time should consider what I wanted to make it clear what I was going to wear to work and also the items of clothes I was going to raid the charity shops for. As the sunrise alarm had woken me up stupidly early, I thought it was a valuable time to make my lunch to carry to work. Plenty of sheep do that so I'm not the wayward sheep sat munching bean falafel in the corner. I'm not alone, Charlene sits next to me for lunch. It has been a competition to come out with the best lunch each day. I've given up competing as I firmly believe she has an advantage with Barry in the background. The dude is getting a TV series for crying out loud. A definite red-card to be given for unfair advantage during the make-believe game I have created to myself. I haven't created a title of this game yet, mostly because I've lost in successive games. I've just fallen down to the title, 'lunch' but I would like it to have a snappier sounding edge.

I looked out to the opposite farm to where the desperate mooing was coming from. The calf was evidently still unwell, and in the hospital as it was only its mother left standing letting out sporadic moos. I saw a vet walk up to her and raised a gun to her forehead, I knew what was going to happen next. When the loud shot ran out, I didn't want the cow to obviously die. However, she did.

Waking up, I felt a large weight hanging over my head and I didn't know why. I definitely didn't do anything to piss them off, in fact they rewarded me with a daily poo. Something I used to struggle with sometimes, in fact, I believed a weekly poo was the norm. So, my mind wandered over what I had ingested – normally the answer I was looking for normally occurred from that thought trail. So that started with my usual breakfast. Porridge oats, no animal lives were lost there. Blueberries did not cause any animals harm so that fitted my vegan diet. I had a packet of crisps, they might not have been vegan. This was something that I learnt from Barry and I didn't believe he would have tricked me. If he has, I need to give a stern word to his girlfriend, Charlene, he promised me that crisps were vegan, my instinct tells me that the packet I ate, was not. Why else would I feel an icky feeling inside of me?

As part of my morning's daily occurrences, my phone buzzed with Charlene's number. I wondered what the daily gossip would be.

"Hey, Shirl! How are you doing? There's nothing much to report on for the gossip front. Have you been in contact with Richard to arrange drinks with him?"

That was a bolt out of the blue. Having had the date of nothingness with Justin and all of the preparations to go with the seldom date, I haven't spent time or effort preparing for the most important date. If I were to mention this to Charlene, then I would get a date. This date would include a shopping trip, accessory buying and probably make-up. This could feasibly happen. After acknowledging this, I should have become excited. However, not a bounce of excitement occurred.

"From your silence, I'm guessing you haven't contacted Richard? I'm sure you would have told me if you did. Isn't that right, Shirl?"

She got me. I was too much of a wimp when it came to anything Richard-related. What was clogging up my mind? It must have been those crisps I ate yesterday. Now was the best chance to discuss Barry's lie of crisps being vegan.

"So, I've been feeling a bit mind cloggy and I've run through what foods I've eaten because normally I can find out exactly what non-vegan food confused me. I've brought it down to the crisps I ate. They were obviously non-vegan."

The loud cacophonic laughter made me pull my ear away from the phone. My dietary finding was not meant to be funny. I waited for over a minute for her to finish laughing before I gave a loud audible sigh.

"Sorry, Shirl, you really crack me up. Crisps are vegan. We've gone over this before with Barry. Although the flavour of the crisps is called 'Smokey Bacon' it will not have been used by a living animal. Its flavours come from scientists that can replicate the same taste. I can ask Barry to talk you through it some more if you like?"

This was annoying. I believed Barry from when he first told us this fact. No offers of food taste tampering is needed from Barry. The crisps knowledge all came flooding back to me.

"So, what else could have disrupted my thinking if I scoffed just vegan food? There must have been something else that happened yesterday that made my mind get itself into a fuddle."

My thoughts acted out where I was in the evening. After work, I went into the kitchen to make a superb stir-fry and thought the horrendous cow screaming would be less if I went to my bedroom. The screaming was much of the same when I sat on my bed. I pulled the curtains aside to look out onto the farm opposite.

"I know why I was in a fuzz! The farmer opposite me brought out a pistol and shot the cow who was mooing. Oh my god, the farmer took the calf away and was probably not going to give it back. So, the farmer just killed her."

Although, I couldn't see Charlene, I could sense she was nodding by giving out lots of 'Uh-huh's'. Finally, things started to fall in place. I could discuss what I witnessed whenever I met Richard. I should start this action by mentioning this to Charlene.

"Okay, Charlene, let's get this Richard date thing going! Can you help in any way?"

Of course, she could. Date preparation was one of her best skills. Having cleared my mind of the brain fog, I decided that I needed to have an excellent date with Richard. I hoped I'd never witness a murder like that again.

The high-street called us like it did before the Justin, no hope, date. The charity shops sang to us as we trotted past them. It didn't take long before I found a sexy slinky dress. Yes, hopefully I'll be able to show off my new veganfied figure.

Charlene agreed to do my make-up, so I felt relaxed with that. Tomorrow is the twenty eighth, when Richard is likely to be around. Thankfully, my time of shopping made my night's slumber easy to attain. I slept like a lamb surrounded by cushions until my sunrise alarm woke me up.

The morning was joyful to endure. Instead of being annoyed, the birdsong was quite uplifting. That was a notion that I've never endured. Normally, the smaller birdies singing was a bit annoying because I'm normally in a grumpy mood. However, today I knew exactly my day's itinerant and it will finally fill my wishes. The only thing I needed was a sultry kiss from Richard. That was not something I was in charge of.

Everything else was prepared to a high standard. Even if I do say so myself.

My phone joined in with all the bird song. My mind was prepared for a date debrief with Charlene as well as any other gossip she felt was important to tell me. It was quite a shock to hear an unexpected male voice. Staying cool was my main thinking to get me through this call. It couldn't be Richard already could it?

"Hey, Shirley, sorry for calling you this early but I just wanted to make sure you're around for a meet later?"

It was then after he said that, when I realised I didn't know the sound of Richard's actual voice. Some other ram could have phoned me. Without wanting to sound overly up myself I asked the question. "Who am I speaking with?" If the gentle ram gave the perfect answer, I decided to squeal.

"I'm sorry for interrupting your morning, I was told you wanted to meet with me. My name's Richard."

A squeal duly took place. Afterwards, I felt a lengthened happy sigh could come out. We decided the noodle bar would be the best place for us to dine. Seeing that we're both vegans. And we're both aware of its location. And we both are looking forward to the new dish we will try next.

'Sorry, Shirley, I can't make tonight. Can you make our date tomorrow?'

Well, that was rubbish. I could, of course, make tomorrow. I won't reply until seven minutes. This matches to his earlier reply to me.

'Sure, let's do tomorrow.'

I consciously omitted a kiss, although I deeply wanted to include one. I didn't want a weak date sign-off. I wanted a passionate love exchange. I hoped Richard felt the same way.

Both Charlene and I fancied a trip to the noodle bar. Mostly, because it was the best vegan place to eat. I know it was a favourite place Richard also frequents, if I were to become acquainted with him, then I would approve.

"Richard! Come here! Shirley and I have dropped in. You should sit with us!"

My love for my new best friend grew deeper. I could be sat on the same table as Richard. His mere presence could fuel his interest in having a date with me. I needed to be on my best behaviour. The sexy glances needed to be kept at a minimum. Difficult task, but I didn't want to scare him off. I needn't have worried for too long, Richard began to speak.

'Shirley, do you fancy coming with me?'

How could I have any other answer than, "Oh right, yes, okay!"

I sensibly waited a couple of moments before answering his question.

'Thanks for your offer. Yes, I would love to sit with you.'

I shouldn't have accepted the table he proposed. It was the same where I sat with Justin. I patted myself on the back in doing so as it made myself seem calm and confident. This was the opposite of how I was feeling. Did my hair look brilliant? I believed in Charlene's skills in the beauty department. I even started to fancy myself when I looked in the mirror, after all it felt as if she if yanked half of my wool out, so I felt the inner need to enter the deep appreciation mode.

The decision I made next, fearing it truly wonderful; Richard was a handsome ram. I know I spent a long time glaring at him when we went to the pub the other night, but now I could glare at his eyes. Without looking odd. Especially when I noticed his eye colour. I was lazy and assumed they were brown. Quite a popular colour but I feel his brown had the edge. There were around seven various shades of brown in his iris which made my departure from the table difficult as the counting of colours was enjoyable to experience.

No, No, No. Richard's ex was sat at the back of the restaurant. How could this happen? I mean there must be other places to go to in this town. Unless, of course, she has decided to turn vegan. This could not be true as Charlene has told me she definitely isn't. I don't believe Charlene could be wrong on this front so that means the ex has come to stalk Richard. I chose to employ my flirting ability to a higher level. If the ex wants to get Richard, she will have to dodge me first.

My eyelashes flickered when I asked if he had been in this restaurant before. I knew he had been as I witnessed him whilst I was on a date with Justin, it would be interesting to hear his answer. He couldn't possibly lie.

"Well, yes actually, this is my favourite restaurant around here." Richard was obviously an honest ram as well as being beautiful, that was not a lie. Okay how about some physical interaction to progress my flirty level.

I rested my right hoof over his leg, nothing sexual just giving him a relaxed emittance from me. This will make him finding love with me easier. This was a plan I couldn't believe would fail. It all happened not long after the leg resting when I saw the ex-migrate herself to the toilets. A good appearance was held by her, I didn't realise floral dresses were quite as popular. My eyes returned to their Richard admiring position. Should I follow the ex to the toilet? Not for anything underhandly. I just wanted to know what she wanted to do tonight.

As I entered the toilets, I could see a flowery make-up bag on the sinks in-front of the mirror. I checked myself out in the mirror, I still look good, and I'm surprised Richard hasn't gone for me already. A toilet door opened and out walked the ex who obviously copied me by checking herself out in the mirror, but she differs by my actions and tuts whilst reaching for her make-up bag. I was surprised that she would give another coat of mascara without noticing of me making a sound. She looked straight at me and I froze as was confused to whether I should say anything. I just looked straight back at her and gave a reluctant smile. To this she burst into speech.

"Hi there, you look familiar. Are you working at Burley Farm?"

Oh dear, I felt the need to answer her question something that I didn't want to be involved in, she was after all the ram who I'm sat with ex-girlfriend. Did she know of this? I suppose I would answer.

"No, I work in Barton Farm. I have seen you around." I thought I'd offer a smile.

"Oh yes, I think I've seen you too, is it Sharon, your name?"

This is annoying, I felt proud she got the first two letters of my name correct at least. This does not mean I should correct her. I am after all wanting to become romantic with her ex. No, I am not saying anything. I will elegantly spin and gracefully exit the toilets.

Once sat down at our table, I offered Richard a gentle smile. We spoke about all sorts of things in the farm life, nothing I didn't already know. One thing I would love to find out is regarding his ex, should I ask anything regarding this?

It didn't take long after thinking this the ex-swishes round and glides her hoof down Richard's back and leg. What an insulting bitch! I thought we had created a good level of appreciation of our standings but obviously not by her doing that.

I looked at how Richard received the unwelcomed rush of inappropriate advances. Thankfully, Richard looked utterly surprised and even raised his eyebrows.

Should I say anything to agree with him? My toilet friend just decided to ruin my date, okay maybe she was being overly nice to her ex. I did not want any interruption to our date.

Once the ex had passed our table, she left with a screech of "See ya!" so I felt a sense of sympathy for the ewe. The feeling of desperation was perfectly demonstrated by her being here. My realisation of Richard sat opposite me was a sudden surprise. He had a large smile and gave a gentle nod. The smile wasn't going anywhere despite his ex squawking at him. I felt honoured to have his stare whilst she darted around him. I hoped he would say something delightful to hear. Possibly, 'do you want to have a drink?' or, 'You're looking gorgeous tonight'; both wonderful statements. I think the overall winner was the alcohol one. That was the moment I missed Charlene the most. I needed a briefing of what had happened so far. Nothing exciting so far, just a bubbling excitement under the skin. An answer was needed to be given.

The night's sleep was far from restful. I looked back on every moment shared with Richard. A collective decision regarding the length of interaction with him couldn't have been more than ten minutes, for the sake of living on this planet, I neglected to have more interaction with him. My mind created plays of doing this; accidentally falling into him, tripping up on a stone close to him, crying out for a farmyard emergency. A standard text could suffice to engage him in conversation. The construction of which would involve Charlene. Probably. My mental neurons flicked to attention, should I mention our meet? Should I ask him about the noodle dish he ate last night? Should I mention the fact I met his ex in the toilet? After replaying all of these thoughts, I realised the best way in going forward will be to not say a peep about last night and rely on myself.

'Hello, Miss Shirley, how are you doing on this fine day?'

Thankfully, my new best friend stepped through my barn doors, she would know how best to answer Richard's text. Enormous appreciation swept over me, thank goodness Richard stepped into our trotting circle first. Charlene proceeded to wildly squeal and hoof clap.

"This is amazing! You obviously didn't do anything upsetting. What are you going to reply with? Do you want me to do it?"

I sat down and sighed. Some group of brain cells were decided the best course of action would be for me to answer myself. With Charlene to check before I clicked sent.

"I thought I would say something like how I had a good time on our date and whether we could continue on another meet. What do you think about that?"

I knew as soon as I said those words, they were perfect to be wrapped up and sent back to him.

'Hi, Mr Richard, I'm having a fine day. I had a great time last night, don't suppose you fancy another meet?'

Pride enveloped all over my body, I had created that message. Admittedly, Charlene had the final glance over my screen before clicking send but she had not changed any of the content and just gave a subtle nod.

All of my pride was stomped over by the swarm of doubt. What if he didn't want to see me again? He seemed like a confident and cool gentle-ram, partly, because he must have been to start on the vegan journey. He may have been part of the sober flock. A group of sheep who do not ingest any alcohol. A notion I could not partake in, largely because I love drinking wine. It clicked with me why sheep say they couldn't possibly go vegan because they loved cheese so much. A notion I learnt a lot about in the recent past, especially the dastardly protein found in dairy. It makes you want to eat more. And more. Casein was the devil.

'Yes, definitely, let's go for a drink!'

Well, that was worth the seven minute wait. I shouted over to Charlene, she must be excited when I read out my new Richard text.

"YES! Darling! I'll arrange the costume. If you want me to."

This was something I knew she was good at, despite making it seem like I was putting on a show by using the word, 'costume' I knew exactly what she meant. I smiled and nodded then proceeded to get excited. Richard wanted to go out with me, and I didn't need to coerce him.

"There's a cool coffee place down the high street actually. Barry and I went to it. You two should definitely go there."

The location was decided as well as what I was wearing, or 'costume' as Charlene puts it. Operation V was good for blast off. The location Charlene specified was a quaint coffee house with a noticeable green sign with the word VEGAN on the front door. This made me feel relaxed. And slightly annoyed I never knew of it being here. Time to find the best seating location. Charlene told me there were cute tables for two at the back, something I could have found by myself.

When I felt the pull of my navigation toward the back, my eyes stumbled upon Richard sat with a bottle of red wine and two glasses in front of him. The smile instantly spread across my face and the realisation of actually meetings the best looking of the farms in my area actually struck, I needed to look cool and calm. When I made eye contact with Richard, I was instantly rewarded with one of his bright smiles. The sort I saw in the pub that night, the moments of magnificence. One was directed at me.

"Hey, Shirley! Great spot!"

He stood up and walked around the table and moved towards giving me a hug. Charlene had trained me well in the art of air kissing, so I employed that tactic. I would come across as pure elegance and class. Richard pulled the bottle of wine toward me. His smile blossomed even more.

"It looks good, a bit surprised they sell wine here though, being a coffee café, but I'd never say no to a glass of wine. Especially as its vegan!"

Richard promptly stood up and looked confused. I wondered if I should say something, I needn't have worried as he started to make a sound. Just a grumble before he asked, "Would you like a coffee?"

What an unexpected statement. My intrigue was captured by the wineglasses and bottle of wine. A pleasant refusal was given regarding coffee, but I thanked him for thinking about me. He offered me a smile. I needed to warm up my vocal chords so asked a question.

"Maybe a coffee first and then if we wanted, we could move on to wine?"

The smile was back, so I ordered a coconut latte. Oat milk Cappuccino was his coffee choice. We both sat down in a similar position to last night by looking at each other. He broke away from the staring by asking a question.

"So how are you finding veganism? It was only a few weeks ago since I saw you with a poorly tummy."

Oh crap, he can remember vomit gate. The only thing I could say is praising plant-based eating and hopefully he'd forget it.

"You went on an eating trip before going vegan. Is that right?"

I felt ashamed to agree, but I did. The Richard smile did not disappear. He told me he did the same thing before turning. This made me feel better although I couldn't quite believe it was true. He was just amazing, I couldn't believe it to be true. He was Mr Vegan to me, I couldn't understand he existed being a carnivore.

"Well, yes. Both Charlene and I went to the doughnut factory in town and decided to eat as many donuts as possible. I know now there are alternatives, I just thought going vegan meant I couldn't have all the nice sweet things. Cakes and donuts being the worst culprits."

I looked up at Richard to see the smile come back accompanied by raised eyebrows.

"I know exactly what you mean, I was in the same spot when I turned vegan. It's so bizarre to think that way now we know how bad food can be."

I thought it best to pour the wine as the bottle was calling me. Richard obviously approved as he pushed his glass in my direction. I thought I'd try out the Gbombs on him, I'd soon see how much he valued being a vegan.

"Have you ever heard of Gbombs?"

The question was put out there. I knew all the information regarding this. Charlene had drummed it into me, probably because of her boyfriend being a vegan rock star. It would be interesting to hear how he would answer.

"Well, yes, actually. Gbombs are the foods you should eat to get the most nutrition, yes?"

My sympathetic smile was given, this could be an interesting conversation. I was a pro regarding this.

"So okay, G stands for greens, yes?"

I felt almost sympathetic, of course, it stands for greens. I should offer the next letters. This would strengthen our bonds in doing so.

"B stands for beans."

He brought back his smile and began to speak.

"Yes, that's right. O stands for onions. M stands for mushrooms."

A glint clearly emitted from him, I wondered if he'd remember what B is. I struggled with that one. It is berries of course.

"Ah, B we've already said beans. Hmmm, what is it? Ah. I'll get it in a second."

Now this felt like I knew the punch line of a joke. He wouldn't want me to ruin him trying to remember. Would he?

"Don't suppose you know what B stands for? Apart from beans."

"B is for berries."

I sat back with a smile and felt relaxed. I was determined not to say anymore.

"Oh, well done, yes you're right. S stands for seeds. I know that."

"Yes, that's right. Well done."

We reverted back to our stare-athon between ourselves, something I really enjoyed. Should I mention meeting his ex in the toilets? Probably not. To tell him about meeting his ex in an unplanned location, could either annoy him or make him fall more in love with me. I should definitely say something. "I met your ex last night in the toilets. I thought I'd say something."

Richard let out a large push of air in surprise. A quizzical look may provoke some words.

"She's a bit muddled. I hope she didn't say anything to upset you."

"She wasn't a bitch, she said she thought my name was Sharon. Nothing much wrong with that."

Richard let out a quick laugh.

"She knows your name, Shirley. She has mentioned you a lot in the past. She thinks you're beautiful and wears good clothes."

Well, this was nice to hear. I thought the same things about her. Why did she think that? She was, after all part of a rival farm. A farm that was full of beautiful ewes.

"Is she a vegan? I know there are many in the Burley Farm."

Richard raised his eyebrows at me and shook his head.

"I wish she was, unfortunately her uncle had a sudden heart attack and died. I just wish she would have been more open with her dietary choices. Going vegan from the start could have nulled any stroke or heart attack risk. She was just too stubborn to contemplate losing cream or cheese. I know it doesn't mean we couldn't go out, but when she mocked me when choosing vegan options, I thought I didn't want to be in this relationship."

A valid point of view. I felt the same way the day I turned vegan. All of the flock smeared at me when I turned vegan. As well as Charlene. Something I hoped Richard recognised. When I looked towards him, I noticed him pouring wine into my glass. I offered a smile to thank him.

"Are you doing anything tonight? As in, do you have any plans?"

My mind wanted to say I wouldn't mind a plan involving him and his bed. It might be too much of a brash thing to say.

"No, do you?"

To my delight, Richard's smile appeared, and he put his hoofs in mine.

"I don't have any plans, but I wouldn't mind a plan involving you."

He said that. Richard actually said that.

I felt it best to try out his kisses. Once I enjoyed his kissing style, I felt it best to say something.

"Let's try out your plan with me then."

I gave him a quick peck on his forehead and smiled. Quite tame compared to our first kiss.

The evening and night were the best I have experienced. Thank you, vegan gods! That sounded a bit twee, even to my standards. It was the truth and my smug head couldn't get any larger.